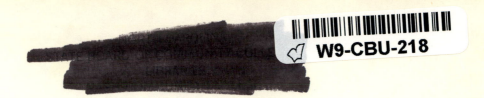

GERMS

Mysterious Microorganisms

These and other books are included in the
Encyclopedia of Discovery and Invention
series:

GERMS
Mysterious Microorganisms

by DON NARDO

The ENCYCLOPEDIA of
D·I·S·C·O·V·E·R·Y
and **INVENTION**

P.O. Box 289011 SAN DIEGO, CA 92198-9011

Library of Congress Cataloging-in-Publication Data

Nardo, Don, 1947-
    Germs: mysterious microorganisms / by Don Nardo.
      p. cm.— (The Encyclopedia of discovery and invention)
    Includes bibliographical references and index.
    Summary: Discusses the nature and function of germs and how they
can be responsible for both good and bad effects.
    ISBN 1-56006-214-2
    1. Microbiology—Juvenile Literature.   [1. Microorganisms.
2. Microbiology.] I. Title.   II. Series.
QR57.N37 1991
616'.01—dc20   91-15569

Printed in the USA

Contents

Foreword

The belief in progress has been one of the dominant forces in Western Civilization from the Scientific Revolution of the seventeenth century to the present. Embodied in the idea of progress is the conviction that each generation will be better off than the one that preceded it. Eventually, all peoples will benefit from and share in this better world. R.R. Palmer, in his *History of the Modern World*, calls this belief in progress "a kind of nonreligious faith that the conditions of human life" will continually improve as time goes on.

For over a thousand years prior to the seventeenth century, science had progressed little. Inquiry was largely discouraged, and experimentation, almost nonexistent. As a result, science became regressive and discovery was ignored. Benjamin Farrington, a historian of science, characterized it this way: "Science had failed to become a real force in the life of society. Instead there had arisen a conception of science as a cycle of liberal studies for a privileged minority. Science ceased to be a means of transforming the conditions of life." In short, had this intellectual climate continued, humanity's future would have been little more than a clone of its past.

Fortunately, these circumstances were not destined to last. By the seventeenth and eighteenth centuries, Western society was undergoing radical and favorable changes. And the changes that occurred gave rise to the notion that progress was a real force urging civilization forward. Surpluses of consumer goods were replacing substandard living conditions in most of Western Europe. Rigid class systems were giving way to social mobility. In nations like France and the United States, the lofty principles of democracy and popular sovereignty were being painted in broad, gilded strokes over the fading canvasses of monarchy and despotism.

But more significant than these social, economic, and political changes, the new age witnessed a rebirth of science. Centuries of scientific stagnation began crumbling before a spirit of scientific inquiry that spawned undreamed of technological advances. And it was the discoveries and inventions of scores of men and women that fueled these new technologies, dramatically increasing the ability of humankind to control nature—and, many believed, eventually to guide it.

It is a truism of science and technology that the results derived from observation and experimentation are not finalities. They are part of a process. Each discovery is but one piece in a continuum bridging past and present and heralding an extraordinary future. The heroic age of the Scientific Revolution was simply a start. It laid a foundation upon which succeeding generations of imaginative thinkers could build. It kindled the belief that progress is possible as long as there were gifted men and women who would respond to society's needs. When Antonie van Leeuwenhoek observed *Animalcules* (little animals) through his high-powered microscope in 1683, the discovery did not end there. Others followed who would call these "little animals" bacteria and, in time, recognize their role in the process of health and disease. Robert Koch, a German bacteriologist and winner of the Nobel Prize in Physiology and Medicine, was one of these men. Koch firmly established that bacteria are responsible for causing infectious diseases. He identified, among others, the causative organisms of anthrax and tuberculosis. Alexander Fleming, another Nobel Laureate, progressed still further in the quest to understand and control bacteria. In 1928, Fleming discovered penicillin, the antibiotic wonder drug. Penicillin, and the generations of antibiotics that succeeded it, have done more to prevent premature death than any other discovery in the history of humankind. And as civilization hastens toward the twenty-first century, most agree that the conquest of van Leeuwenhoek's "little animals" will continue.

The *Encyclopedia of Discovery and Invention* examines those discoveries and inventions that have had a sweeping impact on life and thought in the modern world. Each book explores the ideas that led to the invention or discovery, and, more importantly, how the world changed and continues to change because of it. The series also highlights the people behind the achievements—the unique men and women whose singular genius and rich imagination have altered the lives of everyone. Enhanced by photographs and clearly explained technical drawings, these books are comprehensive examinations of the building blocks of human progress.

GERMS

. . . .

Mysterious Microorganisms

GERMS

Introduction

Before the discovery of germs, people were mystified by the spread of disease. They blamed the unpredictable acts of the gods, the evil influence of supernatural beings, and even their neighbors and friends to explain why a certain plague struck them without warning. It would not even occur to our ancestors that eating rancid food, drinking contaminated water, or failing to wash their hands would be the true cause of many diseases.

Doctors and others who healed the sick and ministered to other health needs were as ignorant as the rest of the population about the existence of germs and the causes of disease. It was not uncommon, for example, for doctors to see dozens of patients each day without ever stopping to wash their hands. This lack of simple hygiene undoubtedly resulted in the spread of countless illnesses and death. Such was the case with childbed, or puerperal fever. Doctors carried the fever germs on their hands from birthing bed to birthing bed. One doctor with dirty hands could spread the disease through an entire hospital ward in a single day. In this way, the disease spread, killing thousands of women.

Had past human societies known that an act as simple as hand washing

■■■ TIMELINE: GERMS

1 ■ 1347
Mongols hurl dead bubonic plague victims into the Italian walled city of Kaffa, spreading the disease in Europe.

2 ■ 1590
Zacharias Janssen builds the first compound, or two-lensed, microscope.

3 ■ 1673
Antonie van Leeuwenhoek discovers the existence of germs.

4 ■ 1767
Lazzaro Spallanzani performs experiments suggesting that germs do not spontaneously come to life.

5 ■ 1854
Louis Pasteur discovers that germs cause fermentation and food spoilage.

6 ■ 1861
Pasteur disproves the theory of spontaneous generation.

7 ■ 1864
Dr. Joseph Lister begins using antiseptics.

8 ■ 1876
Robert Koch proves the germ theory of disease.

could halt the spread of some diseases, life might have been very different. Unfortunately, it would take the discovery of germs and their relationship to disease to change people's habits. This discovery, when it finally came, was nothing short of miraculous. For the first time in human history, scientists realized that people might not be so helpless in the face of disease. Researchers devoted hundreds of hours to learning about germs and their links to disease. Most importantly, perhaps, researchers learned that simple hygiene would go a long way toward preventing the growth and spread of many harmful germs. In hospitals, for example, sanitation standards and practices, sometimes as simple as routinely changing and washing bedsheets were introduced.

Ultimately, the discovery of germs would lead to other phenomenal discoveries, including vaccines and antibiotics. These discoveries are covered in other books in the Discovery and Invention Series. But for any of these remarkable inventions to happen, it took a combination of luck, study, and scientific curiosity to bring about the most primary discovery of all: that within our world, there is another world filled with thousands of mysterious, microscopic organisms that affect us in countless ways. It is this story that unfolds in *Germs: Mysterious Microorganisms*.

9 ■ 1892
First experiments conducted suggesting the existence of viruses.

10 ■ 1918
Huge influenza epidemic sweeps the world.

11 ■ 1925
Many nations sign the Geneva Protocol, promising not to build and use biological weapons.

12 ■ 1939
Japan opens the world's first biological weapons testing facility.

13 ■ 1972
Eighty-seven nations sign the Biological Warfare Convention, banning the use of germ weapons.

14 ■ 1989
First major use of germs to clean up an oil spill, the *Exxon Valdez* disaster in Alaska's Prince William Sound.

15 ■ 1991
The U.S. and its allies identify and bomb Iraq's biological weapons facilities during the Persian Gulf War.

CHAPTER 1

Trying to Explain the Ravages of Disease

Before people knew about germs, the chances of catching a disease and dying from it were much greater than they are today. No one realized that millions of germs swarmed everywhere—in the air people breathed, the water they drank, the food they ate, the soil they tilled, and even on their own bodies. Dangerous germs passed freely from person to person, from house to house, and from village to village. As a result, periodic outbreaks of crippling or deadly diseases have occurred throughout history. Epidemics of measles, yellow fever, bubonic plague, leprosy, cholera, typhus, smallpox, and other maladies regularly wiped out thousands or millions of people at a time. The horrors associated with these plagues were accepted as facts of life in every culture.

Living with Filth and Decay

For thousands of years, most people lived in filthy, unsanitary conditions. They did not like the way they lived, but they did not know any better. Many families lived in stone or wooden shacks, with as many as six to ten people living in one or two rooms. Many of these dwellings had cold dirt floors, which turned damp and soggy when it rained. Sleeping and eating areas often became caked with mud from the outside and littered with decaying scraps of food from the inside.

Those who lived in nicer houses with wooden floors were not much better off. They, too, were exposed to the garbage that most people threw into the streets, walkways, and gardens. Germs grew in the rotting garbage. People and animals then walked on this litter and carried the germs into houses on their shoes or feet.

The streets also bore signs of human and animal waste. Some people kept buckets or barrels for these wastes in the house. When these containers

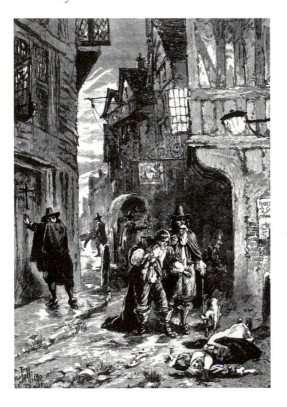

An eighteenth-century woodcut depicts life in London in the 1650s as filthy, crowded, and unsanitary.

the water, contaminating it as they went.

Most people were also careless in preparing the food they ate. They often slaughtered their animals with dirty knives, then stored the meat in hot, filthy cellars. Few people washed vegetables and fruits before eating them. Often, people ate fruits and vegetables that insects and rodents had nibbled. Refrigeration did not exist. Without refrigeration, which slows the growth of germs, food did not keep very long before it spoiled. Vegetables lasted a few days at most, but people kept meat for weeks, sometimes even months. Germs bred in the spoiled food, and those people who

In the sixteenth century, many people often used a single well for washing clothes and for drinking.

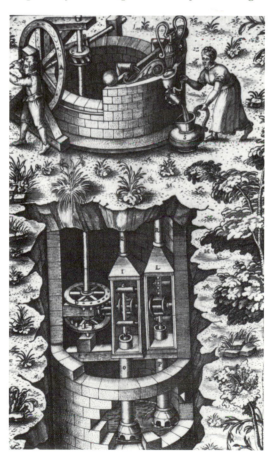

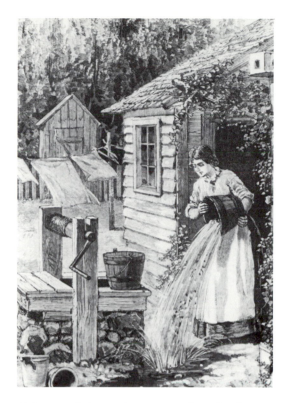

Before people knew about germs, they often kept body and household wastes in buckets. When the buckets were full, people simply dumped them outside, often near their water supplies.

became full, people dumped the wastes into street gutters, backyard manure piles, ponds, and streams. Those with separate outhouses also dumped their accumulated wastes outside in piles. Often, the sun dried the manure into a powder, which the wind blew over villages and houses and into open windows.

It was common for all the inhabitants of a village to use a single well or other water source for both washing clothes and drinking. Most people were not careful about keeping the water clean, and it often became contaminated by garbage, waste, and other litter. In addition, dogs, pigs, goats, and other animals drank from or walked through

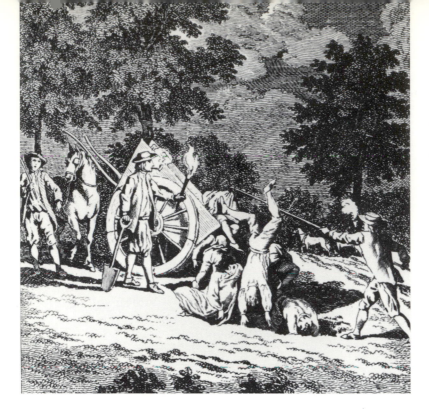

Men handle corpses with their bare hands during an eighteenth-century mass burial. They did not know that decaying corpses can spread disease.

ate it became ill. Often, people did not thoroughly clean their dishes, cups, and knives after eating. The remaining crusts of decaying food were another breeding ground for disease germs.

The decaying corpses of humans and animals also spread diseases. In ancient and medieval times, it was common practice for people to touch rotting bodies with their bare hands while moving and preparing them for burial. In this way, disease traveled from the dead to the living. Sometimes, diseased bodies were thrown into lakes or streams, contaminating the water.

A Widespread Lack of Hygiene

Personal cleanliness was another problem. For the most part, bathing was not a regular habit before the twentieth century. There were exceptions to this rule. For instance, the nobility and

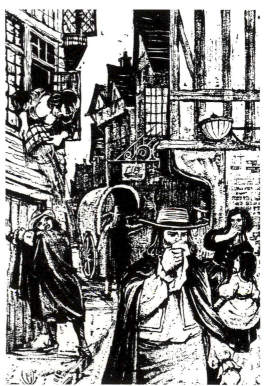

When the bubonic plague swept through London in the 1660s, the dead bodies of plague victims became a common sight on city streets.

wealthy classes in ancient Egypt appear to have bathed frequently. They also covered their freshly washed bodies with special ointments and deodorants. The Romans too placed a great deal of emphasis on cleaning themselves and regularly visited one of the many public baths found in Roman cities. In most cultures, however, personal cleanliness was largely neglected and sometimes actually frowned upon.

The thirteenth-century Christian monk Saint Francis of Assisi proclaimed that refusing to bathe was a gesture that proved one's devotion to God. Many people in Europe followed his teachings and never washed. Spain's Queen Isabella, who granted Columbus his ships, bragged that she had bathed only twice in her life. The first time, she said, was when she was born, the second just prior to her marriage. In colonial Pennsylvania and Virginia, where nudity was viewed as sinful, there were written laws that banned or strictly limited bathing. One law stated that a person who took a bath more than once a month would be jailed.

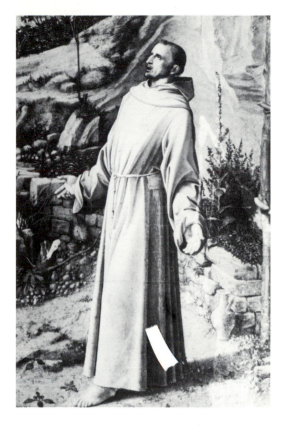

Saint Francis of Assisi, a thirteenth-century Christian monk, refused to bathe to prove his devotion to God. By punishing the flesh, Assisi believed that he would focus more on the spiritual and decry his bodily needs.

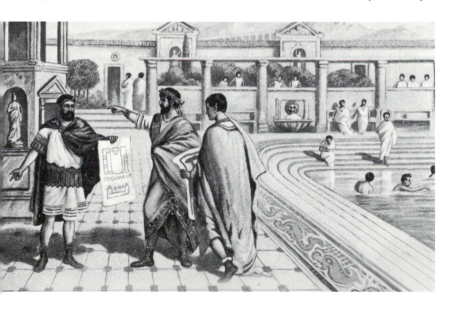

Before the twentieth century, bathing was not a regular habit in most parts of the world. The Romans, however, placed a great deal of emphasis on personal cleanliness. They built and maintained many public baths.

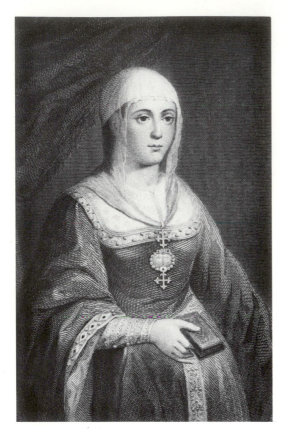

Queen Isabella of Spain bragged that she had bathed only twice in her life—once at birth and once before she married.

Often, being dirty was not just a matter of custom or personal choice. Sometimes, it was difficult to find the proper means to keep clean. Dr. V.W. Greene, an expert on the spread of disease, described the lack of opportunities for bathing in early Great Britain: "There was no running water, streams were cold and polluted, heating fuel was expensive, and soap was hard to get. There just weren't facilities for personal hygiene. Cleanliness wasn't a part of the folk culture [everyday beliefs and habits]."

The consequences of this general lack of hygiene were sometimes disastrous. The dirtier people were, the easier it was for germs and disease to spread. According to Greene, "Europeans and Americans lived in wretched filth, and many died young of associated diseases." Dysentery, childbed fever, and infantile diarrhea killed millions of people in Europe in the nineteenth century alone.

To make matters worse, filthy bodies were, more often than not, infested with bugs. Head lice, bedbugs, fleas,

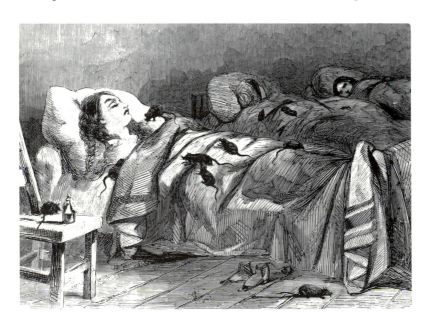

An engraving from Harper's Weekly *depicts conditions in Bellevue Hospital in New York in the 1800s. Even in hospitals, disease-carrying rodents and insects ran rampant.*

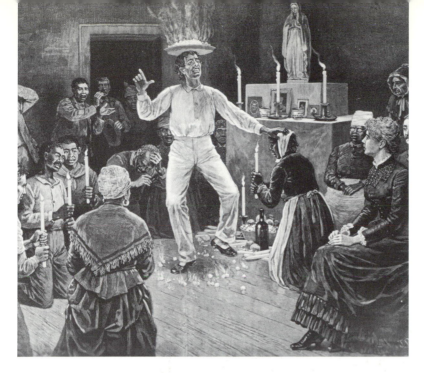

People once believed disease was caused by demons or evil spirits. Here, a man performs a voodoo dance to chase away those spirits.

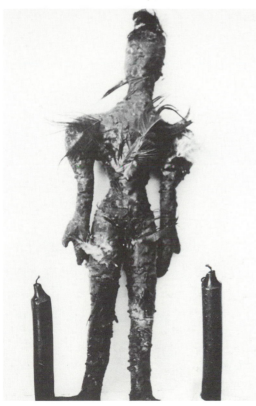

Throughout history, many people thought sorcery, or black magic, caused disease. Some people believed that sorcerers caused illness by stabbing or burning dolls that represented specific people.

and other tiny creatures were unwanted but frequent visitors in most households. More than just irritating pests, these bugs carried deadly diseases. For example, lice often carried relapsing fever, and fleas spread bubonic plague. Infected pests also lived on people's clothes, bed linens, and pets, making it all the more difficult for people to escape the ravages of disease.

Early Beliefs About Disease

Throughout history, people living in such dismal conditions sought explanations for their misery. But because their scientific knowledge of the world was limited, they did not usually find the right answer to their questions.

Early theories about the cause of disease varied from society to society, but most views fell into a few broad categories. One of the most popular beliefs was that disease was the result of sorcery, or black magic. Those who ac-

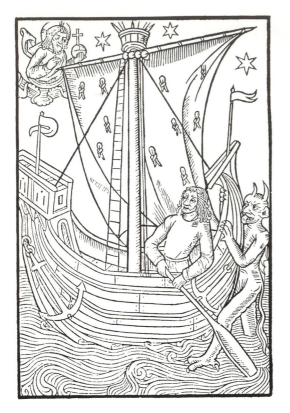

This fifteenth-century woodcut depicts how many people believed that God and the devil controlled many aspects of their lives.

disease was caused by demons or evil spirits that invaded a person's body. Since most people believed that gods and spirits controlled many aspects of their lives, it was natural for them to assume that such spirits were also responsible for disease.

In many cultures, a separate demon existed for each disease. The ancient Mesopotamians, for instance, believed that the demon Ashakku caused consumption, or tuberculosis. Nergal, another mean spirit, brought fever. The worst illnesses were thought to be inflicted by the "evil seven" demons of disease. Mesopotamian doctors were so terrified of these creatures that they became superstitious about the number seven. For example, these doctors refused to treat a patient on the seventh

cepted this supernatural explanation for illness were convinced that sorcerers used magical powers to make people sick.

People believed that one way sorcerers caused illness was by first constructing a doll that represented the victim. When the sorcerer stabbed or burned the doll, the victim supposedly felt the pain. The doll could also be painted or manipulated to make it appear diseased. Then, the victim contracted the disease. Sorcerers could also hurt someone by casting a spell over a discarded remnant from the victim. This remnant might be a hair, a nail clipping, or a piece of excrement.

Some ancient peoples thought that

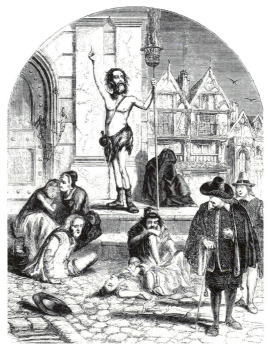

This etching titled "The Great Plague" shows the misery in Europe during the seventeenth century, when an epidemic of bubonic plague swept across the land.

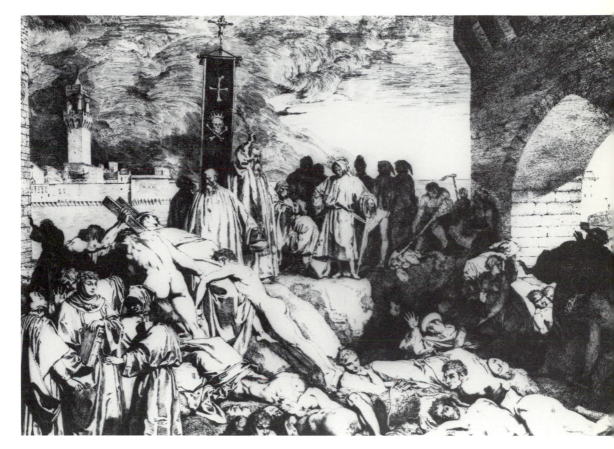

The death toll from the European bubonic plague may have reached twenty-five million people. Here, people in Florence, Italy, prepare to bury plague victims.

day of an illness. They believed that the only cure for a person possessed by a demon was to exorcise, or chase away, the demon.

The Wrath of the Gods

Perhaps the most widespread theory of disease was that it was a punishment brought by the gods. In the most primitive societies, sickness was considered the punishment when someone broke the social or religious taboos. A taboo is a societal rule forbidding people to act in a certain way. Many cultures have taboos against eating certain foods, en-

tering specified areas, and marrying specific kinds of people. Breaking a taboo, many ancients believed, made the gods angry. The punishment might be the infliction of some terrible disease. Belief in taboos was so strong that those who survived the punishment usually never repeated the deed a second time.

In many societies, this concept developed into the idea that a god or gods used disease to punish wicked people. If a person or family caught a disease, it was often considered a sign that someone in the family had angered the gods. When an epidemic spread through a whole town or country, it meant that God believed the entire town or coun-

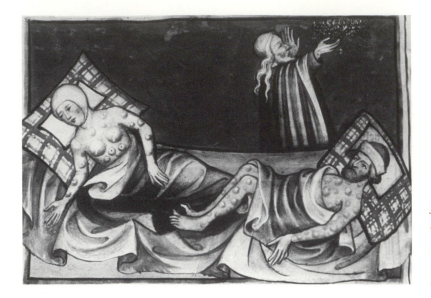

This print from the Toggenburg Bible shows two people suffering from the deadly bubonic plague. During the Middle Ages, the plague killed about one-third of the population of Europe.

try to be corrupt.

The most dramatic example of the belief in disease as punishment was the terrifying outbreak of bubonic plague that occurred in Europe in the fourteenth century. Also called the black death, the plague swept from town to town and from country to country, spreading fear and chaos as well as death. Estimates vary for the overall death toll from the disease. It may have been as high as twenty-five million, almost one-third the population of Europe. No one seemed safe from the black death, which claimed at least one member of nearly every family.

The plague was caused by germs that were carried by fleas. The fleas passed the germs to rats and other animals, which, in turn, brought them to human

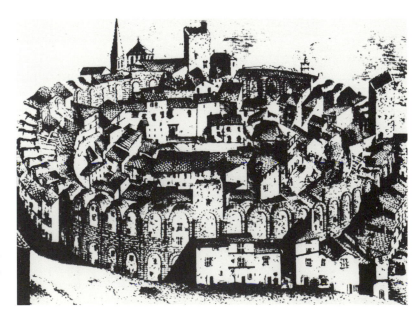

Poor and crowded living conditions contributed to the spread of disease in the Middle Ages.

beings. Of course, this entire process was unknown to people at the time. Most assumed that humanity was finally paying the price for centuries of sin and immorality.

According to religious authorities, the only way to stop the plague was to seek God's forgiveness. At first, people attempted to atone for their sins by praying. It soon became clear that this was not enough, and many people resorted to more desperate measures. Some joined groups of religious fanatics known as flagellants. The flagellants traveled from town to town and attempted to convince people to repent for their sins. Setting themselves up as examples, the flagellants publicly stripped, then beat themselves and each other with spike-tipped whips. They hoped

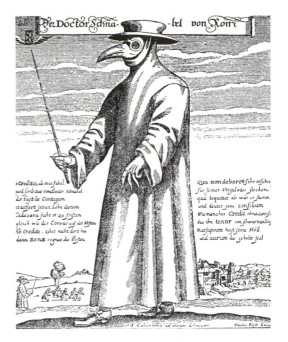

Some people believed that vapors in the air caused disease. Here, a plague doctor wears a mask and clothing designed to protect him from these "bad vapors."

that other people would join them, and some did. They believed that God would eventually see their self-punishment and end the plague.

Rational Explanations

A few people, mostly doctors and scholars, did not accept the idea that the plague was a divine punishment. They correctly believed that the disease was a natural occurrence. One indication was that when people with the plague came into physical contact with healthy people, many of the healthy people contracted the disease. This led these observers to believe that the disease spread when "bad vapors" passed from person to person through the air. Although they did not believe the plague was a divine punishment, their theories of how

Flagellants, like the man shown in this fifteenth-century woodcut, beat themselves publicly to repent for the sins that they believed caused disease.

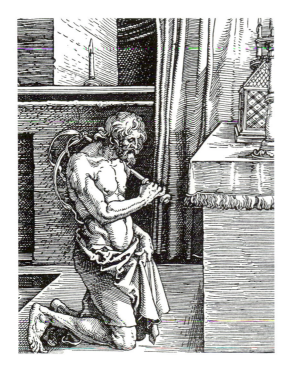

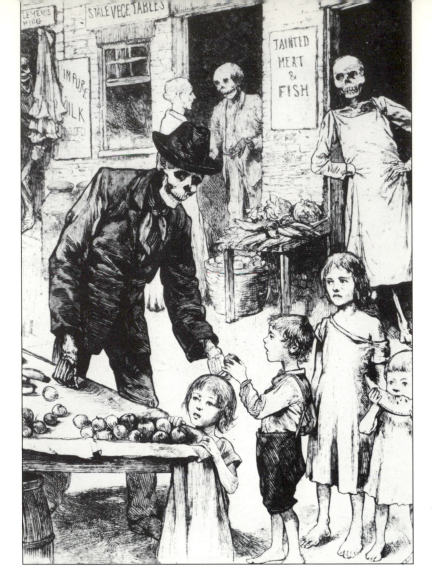

This 1864 print is titled "A hint to the Board of Health on how the city invites the Cholera." It indicates that some people were beginning to link unsanitary conditions with disease, even before the discovery of germs.

the plague and other diseases originated were incorrect. They thought that disease came from poisonous clouds or appeared when the atmosphere changed as the result of influences from stars and planets.

Through the ages, doctors and scientists tried desperately to understand what caused the various diseases that plagued humanity. But people were limited in their discovery of the correct explanation by their lack of technology. Germs are so tiny that they are invisbile to the unaided eye. Advanced medical instruments did not exist, and without devices enabling them to actually see germs, people simply had no way of discovering the existence of these agents of disease. For centuries, the microscopic world of germs—a realm teeming with life—remained hidden from humanity.

Viewing the Mysterious Microscopic World

The invention of the microscope opened the way for the discovery of germs. No one is certain who made the first microscope. Several Europeans built primitive magnifying instruments in the late 1500s and early 1600s. Most of these were simple microscopes that used only one lens. The first person to construct a microscope with two lenses, called a compound microscope, was the Dutch eyeglass maker Zacharias Janssen in 1590.

But none of these early devices were very powerful. They were certainly not powerful enough to reveal organisms as tiny as germs. And better microscopes did not develop very quickly because most people regarded the devices as a novelty. No one considered microscopes to be instruments useful for serious scientific research. Lens makers and others continued to work with their microscopes as a hobby.

A Mouth Filled with Animals

One microscope hobbyist was Antonie van Leeuwenhoek, the owner of a dry goods shop in Delft, in the Netherlands. In addition to running his shop, van Leeuwenhoek also did surveying work and served as Delft's official wine taster. All these duties left him little time for his

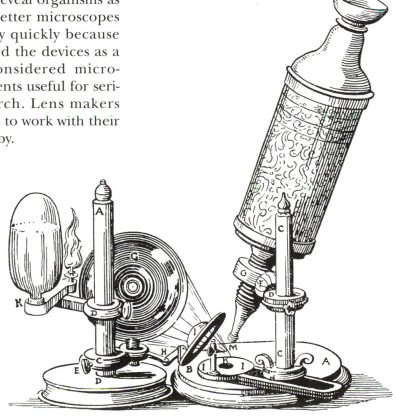

The invention in the sixteenth century of the compound microscope led to the eventual discovery of germs. It enabled scientists to view things that were too small to see with the naked eye.

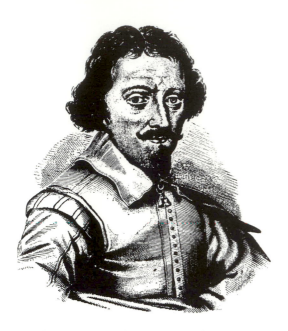

In 1590, Dutch eyeglass maker Zacharias Janssen constructed the first compound microscope.

hobby of grinding glass into fine, polished lenses and using them as magnifying glasses. Because van Leeuwenhoek could devote only a few hours a week to his lenses, his work progressed slowly during the late 1660s and early 1670s.

Eventually, van Leeuwenhoek designed and built his own microscopes. The most advanced of these devices could magnify objects three hundred times, making it much more powerful than other microscopes in use at that time. At first, van Leeuwenhoek observed everyday objects under his microscopes. He looked at hairs, leaves, salt crystals, the eyes and wings of insects, and even specimens of his own blood. All the while, he kept careful notes, describing in detail everything he saw.

In 1673, van Leeuwenhoek noticed what appeared to be tiny creatures swimming in some of the liquids he was studying. He had no idea what these creatures might be. Since they looked and moved like animals, he called them animalcules. Sometimes, he humorously referred to them as "little beasties." In one of his early descriptions of the animalcules, van Leeuwenhoek reported that the creatures were "moving very prettily; some of 'em a bit bigger, others

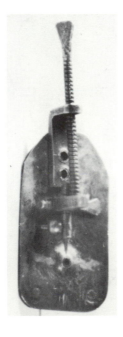

Dutch microscope hobbyist Antonie van Leeuwenhoek was one of the first people to notice tiny creatures swimming in liquid samples under his microscope. At left, is one of his earliest microscopes.

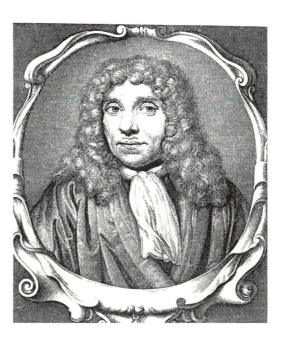

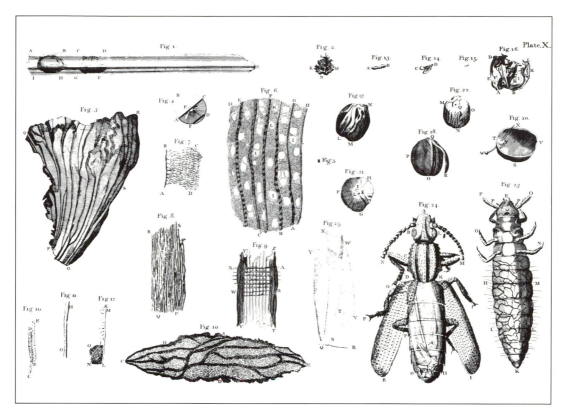

Van Leeuwenhoek used his microscope to look at everyday objects, including hairs, leaves, and insects. He made careful notes and drew pictures (above) of what he saw.

a bit less, than a blood-globule [blood drop]; but all of one and the same make. Their bodies are somewhat longer than broad, and their belly, which was flatlike, furnished with sundry [various types of] little paws . . . they made a quick motion with their paws, yet for all that they made but slow progress."

Van Leeuwenhoek noticed the animalcules in more and more of the substances he studied. He found them in pond water, in food, in urine and excrement, and on the bodies of insects. He also saw vast swarms of the mysterious creatures in the scrapings from between his own teeth. In 1683, van Leeuwenhoek wrote, "For my part I judge . . . that all the people living in our United Netherlands are not as many as the living animals that I carry in my own mouth this very day."

Organisms Without a Purpose?

From 1674 until his death in 1723, van Leeuwenhoek wrote long, detailed letters to the Royal Society of London, a respected organization of British scientists. In the letters, he described his microscopic observations, including those of the animalcules. He also shared this knowledge with other European scholars. But neither van Leeuwenhoek nor any of the other researchers had the slightest idea what the microscopic animals were or where they came from. They certainly did not associate these creatures with disease.

As far as anyone could tell, these microscopic organisms were perfectly harmless and served no particular purpose. To most scientists, the animalcules were curiosities, undeserving of costly and time-consuming study. For more than a century, the few scientists who did study animalcules, which became popularly known as germs during this period, merely cataloged them. The researchers did not offer any important theories about the function germs might serve in nature.

Another reason that knowledge of germs progressed so slowly was the lack of good microscopes. Van Leeuwenhoek's lenses were by far the best of his day, but few people used them. Although van Leeuwenhoek graciously shared most of his discoveries with other scholars, he was very secretive about his work with lenses. He never told anyone how he ground the glass so perfectly, and he never revealed the secret process he used to light his specimens under the microscope. This process was not rediscovered until nearly two centuries later. As a result, few researchers had the technology needed to study germs in any detail until the 1800s.

Life That Sprang from Nowhere

During the late 1600s and all through the 1700s, scientists continued to believe that germs played no vital role in nature. Although there was little or no serious study of germs, the existence of these tiny animals did cause some mem-

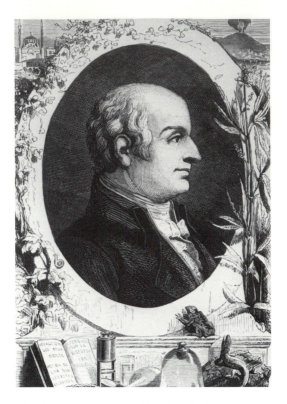

Unlike other scientists of his day, Italian scientist Lazzaro Spallanzani did not believe that life sprang from nonliving matter.

bers of the scientific community to wonder where they came from. This question rekindled a debate that had raged, on and off, for more than a century.

Most scientists believed that life sprang suddenly from nonliving matter. This was called the theory of spontaneous generation. There seemed to be ample evidence for this theory. For example, maggots appeared to grow spontaneously from decaying meat. Rotting wheat produced mice, while toads and snakes appeared from moist soil and mud.

A few scientists disagreed, saying that life could not spring from nonliving materials. They insisted that all living things came from other living things. They argued that maggots appeared in decaying meat because flies had earlier laid eggs in the meat.

Many researchers believed that the existence of germs supported the theory of spontaneous generation. To illustrate their point, the researchers conducted a simple experiment. They observed some water under a microscope and noted the germs floating around in the liquid. They then boiled the water, and the germs disappeared. After a day or two, they looked at the water again. The liquid once more swarmed with the tiny organisms. It appeared that germs had sprung spontaneously into existence from nothing more than everyday water.

An Italian scientist named Lazzaro Spallanzani disagreed with this suggestion. In 1767, he conducted his own experiment with germs. He poured chicken broth teeming with germs into three flasks. He left one flask open, stopped the second with a porous cork, and sealed the third flask completely by melting the glass together at the top. Then, he boiled the broth in each flask, destroying the germs. Within a day, germs reappeared in the first two flasks. But the flask that had been securely sealed remained germ-free.

According to Spallanzani, the experiment proved that germs had entered the boiled broth in the first flask from the air. Because they were so tiny, the germs also penetrated the porous cork in the second flask. But the air and the germs it carried could not get into the third, sealed flask at all, and that was why it was germ-free. Germs did not appear out of nowhere, Spallanzani said. They simply passed unseen through the air.

Spallanzani's experiment did not end the debate over spontaneous generation, but it did shed new light on the behavior of germs. Spallanzani's experiments demonstrated some of the ways in which germs could spread to various materials. Unfortunately, scientists continued to assume that germs, which they began to refer to as microorganisms or microbes, were harmless. They saw no indication that the tiny creatures had any effect whatsoever on either living or nonliving things.

Seeking the Spoilage Culprit

The discovery that germs do bring about changes in other things came quite by accident. In 1854, the well-known French chemist Louis Pasteur received an unusual request. Some French wine

French chemist Louis Pasteur discovered that germs cause changes in other things. His experiments showed that both fermentation and food spoilage were caused by germs.

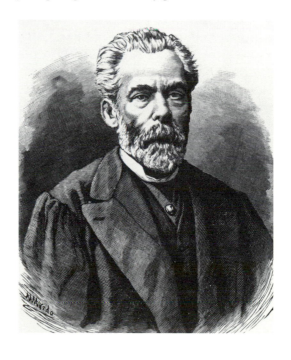

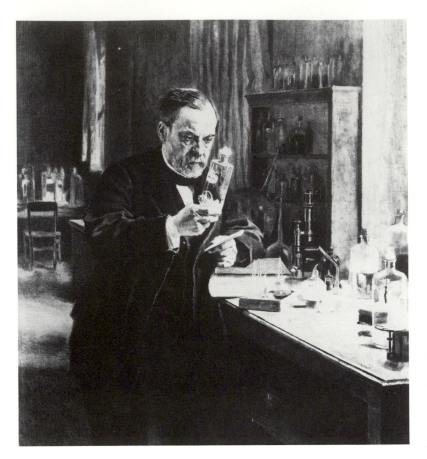

Pasteur conducts one of his many experiments. He created an uproar in the world's scientific community when he showed that yeasts cause fermentation in wine.

makers asked him to find out why their wine was spoiling. Pasteur observed samples of the wine, both spoiled and unspoiled, under his microscope. He noticed large numbers of oval-shaped germs that scientists called yeasts in both batches. He also saw some smaller, rod-shaped germs called bacteria in the spoiled wine. These germs had been seen many times before. The common belief was that they came into existence during the process of fermentation, which changes grape juice into wine by producing alcohol. Scientists thought that during fermentation germs formed as a harmless by-product.

While examining the wine, Pasteur suddenly had a new idea that perhaps not all germs were harmless. Perhaps,

thought Pasteur, germs were causing the wine to spoil. In addition, Pasteur reasoned that the germs might also be the agents that turned the juice into wine. If this were the case, germs were not the result of fermentation, as everyone thought, but rather the cause of the process.

Pasteur Creates an Uproar

To test his assumption, or hypothesis, Pasteur heated mixtures of grape juice and yeasts until the yeasts had been killed. He noted that the grape juice did not change into wine. When he added yeasts to the juice, it fermented normally. This proved conclusively that

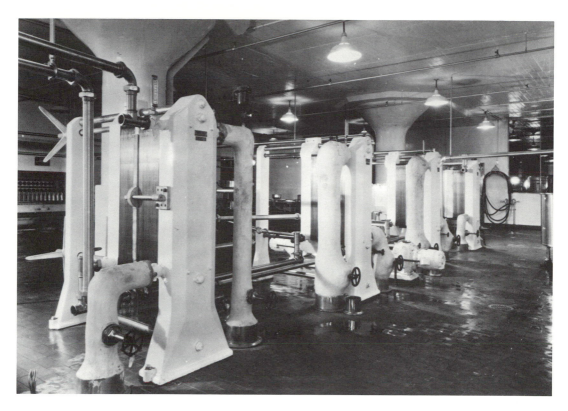

Today, milk and other products are heated quickly in large vats to rid them of harmful bacteria. This process is known as pasteurization, after Louis Pasteur.

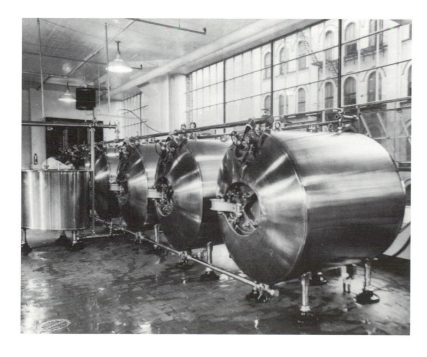

Pasteurization holding tanks.

yeasts caused fermentation. Pasteur noticed that as long as the wine stayed sealed and none of the rod-shaped bacteria entered, it did not spoil. Yet when he added some of the bacteria to the wine, the liquid promptly spoiled. This indicated that some germs caused fermentation, while others produced spoilage.

Pasteur solved the spoilage problem in a simple manner. He heated the wine to a temperature that killed the bacteria but not the yeasts. The wine retained most of its distinctive flavor but did not spoil. In his honor, this heating process became known as pasteurization. A few years later, dairies began pasteurizing milk in order to remove potentially harmful bacteria.

Pasteur's discovery that germs caused fermentation and spoilage created an uproar in the world scientific community. He had shown that germs had specific functions in nature after all. They caused chemical changes in plant juices, and some of these changes were clearly damaging. Other researchers then suggested that germs might also damage animals and people. Scientists in several countries began talking about the possibility that germs actually cause disease.

But there was still a great deal of opposition to this idea in the scientific community. Pasteur realized that it would be difficult to prove beyond question that there was a connection between germs and disease. When, in 1859, his daughter Jeanne died of typhoid fever, Pasteur worked harder than ever to expose the dangers of contact with germs. He believed that it was possible not only to understand the relationship between germs and disease but also to conquer disease.

Establishing the Connection Between Germs and Disease

During the second half of the nineteenth century, the study of germs became known as microbiology. The period between 1854, when Pasteur showed the relationship between germs and fermentation, and 1914 is now referred to as the golden age of microbiology. During these years, scientists made numerous advances in understanding the different types of germs, their structure, and how they behaved. Researchers also proved that germs cause certain diseases and demonstrated how some of these diseases spread.

It was in the late 1850s that Pasteur and other scientists set out to prove that germs cause disease. This concept quickly became known as the germ theory of disease. At the time, the germ theory was very hard for most people to accept. It refuted the traditional explanations that were often intertwined with religious beliefs. For many people, accepting the germ theory would have meant questioning religious truths and values.

There was another reason for the widespread reluctance to accept the germ theory. It did not seem logical. Most people found it extremely hard to believe that invisible creatures could travel through the air and infect plants, animals, and humans. To them, God's wrath seemed a much more believable explanation for disease than germs. Even many scientists refused to accept the idea that such tiny organisms could be responsible for destructive disease.

The theory that germs cause disease was difficult for most people to accept. Instead, people believed God, depicted here creating the earth, caused disease to punish people for their sins.

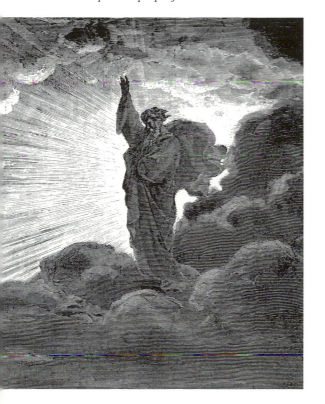

Cells That Come from Other Cells

Pasteur's demonstration that germs cause fermentation and spoilage was the first important step in proving that germs cause disease. His discovery showed that there is a link between the activity of germs and the chemical changes in natu-

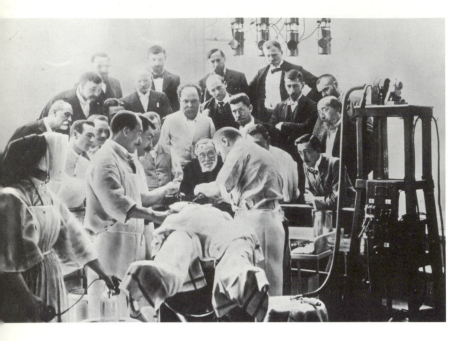

Although German scientist Rudolf Virchow knew that disease was not a magic force, he did not fully understand how it spread. Here, Virchow participates in a skull operation. Simple sanitary techniques—wearing protective gloves and masks—were not employed.

ral substances. Pasteur now attempted to find similar links between germs and disease. He believed that bacteria and other types of germs existed by the trillions in the air and soil and on living things. He proposed that they somehow reproduced and then spread through the environment. Pasteur reasoned that understanding how germs reproduced and spread might lead to ways of controlling them. In this way, disease might also be controlled.

Unfortunately, Pasteur kept encountering resistance from other scientists. They insisted that germs did not reproduce naturally, as plants and animals did. Opponents of the germ theory supported the idea of spontaneous generation, declaring that germs just appeared in random places at random times. Because the existence and behavior of germs were random and unpredictable, they could never be controlled, these scientists said.

Pasteur and other supporters of the germ theory realized that in order to be

taken seriously, they would have to disprove the theory of spontaneous generation. In 1858, the German scientist Rudolf Virchow published an official challenge to spontaneous generation. He proposed the idea of biogenesis, that living cells could come only from other living cells that already existed. Cells are the basic units of living matter from which all plants and animals are built. Germs, which appeared to be one-celled creatures, were produced by other germs, according to this theory. Virchow suggested that cells give rise to new cells by dividing in half.

The biogenesis theory also offered an explanation of how germs are related to disease. Virchow argued that disease is not a magic or divine force that takes hold of a body or body part. Instead, disease begins in the body's cells. Some foreign substance causes cells either to die or to function improperly. Pasteur agreed with Virchow and pointed out that germs are tiny enough to infect the cells of plants and animals. Pasteur

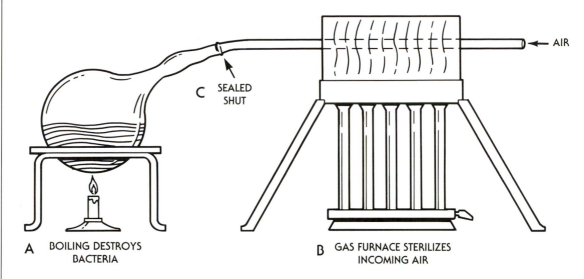

PASTEUR'S EARLY EXPERIMENT

C SEALED SHUT

AIR

A BOILING DESTROYS BACTERIA

B GAS FURNACE STERILIZES INCOMING AIR

The French chemist Louis Pasteur demonstrated that germs did not just suddenly appear but that they are present in the air.

In one of his early experiments, Pasteur placed a liquid teeming with bacteria in a swan-neck flask. He then boiled the liquid and succeeded in destroying the bacteria (A). At the same time, Pasteur used a gas furnace to heat the air entering the flask. The heat killed the bacteria in the incoming air (B). When the flask cooled, Pasteur sealed it shut (C). He found that as long as the flask remained sealed, bacteria could not enter it and contaminate the liquid.

suggested that germs might be the disease-causing foreign substance that Virchow described.

Arguments about biogenesis and spontaneous generation continued until 1861. Fed up with these arguments, Pasteur set up an experiment to clearly show that germs do not arise spontaneously. He repeated the same experiment that Spallanzani had conducted in the 1700s, heating flasks of broth that teemed with germs. But Pasteur's experiment was more carefully controlled than the earlier version. It left no doubt that germs from the air contaminated the broth and multiplied in it and that germs could travel through the air on dust particles. And the experiment illustrated another important point. The fact that some flasks remained germ-free showed that germs could be controlled. With this experiment, Pasteur refuted the idea of spontaneous generation once and for all. The way was now clear for serious microbiology research.

The Germ Theory in Medical Practice

While Pasteur, Virchow, and other scientists sought evidence that germs cause disease, a British surgeon named

Joseph Lister decided not to wait for proof. Lister heard about Pasteur's work in the mid-1860s and agreed that the germ theory made sense. Lister reasoned that if germs move through the air and fall into broth and wine, they might also fall into and infect open wounds.

Lister also remembered what had happened in an Austrian maternity hospital in the late 1840s. A young doctor named Ignaz Semmelweis was disturbed by the high death rate from childbed fever among the women in the hospital's maternity wards. He studied the doctors' daily routines, looking for clues to the problem. He noticed that doctors who worked with corpses in one section of the facility often treated women in the wards immediately afterward. Semmelweis noted that the doc-

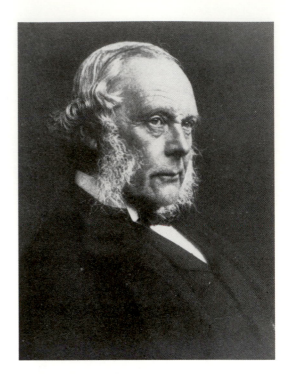

British surgeon Joseph Lister, a believer in Pasteur's germ theory, thought that if doctors used simple sanitary techniques, they could prevent the spread of disease.

tors did not wash their hands after handling the corpses.

As an experiment, Semmelweis asked the physicians to wash with a chlorine rinse before touching the patients. Within a few months, the incidence of childbed fever in the wards decreased dramatically. Semmelweis did not suspect that germs were involved and had no idea what caused the disease. But his experiment suggested that sanitary techniques could help keep disease from spreading. Unfortunately, most doctors at that time considered the experiment a fluke and the results unreliable. They continued to use unsanitary methods.

But Semmelweis's work proved important after all. It influenced Lister, who felt that it supported Pasteur's

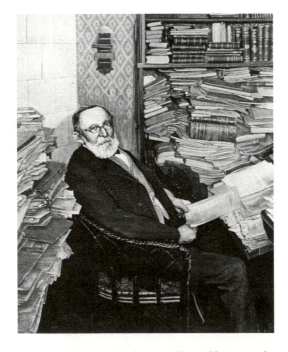

Virchow believed that living cells could come only from other living cells. This theory would later be applied to understanding how germs caused disease.

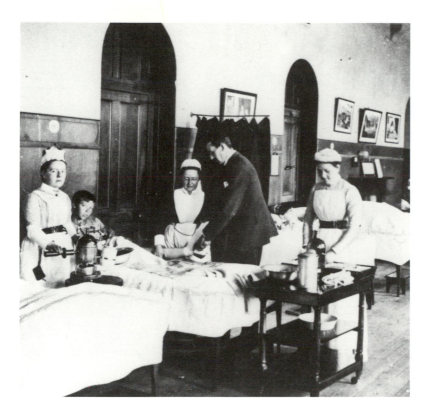

At this hospital in Glasgow, Scotland, Lister first used carbolic acid as an antiseptic in 1864.

ideas about germs and disease. If germs did kill people, thought Lister, there was no time to lose. While Pasteur and other scientists searched for proof of the germ theory, millions of people might be dying needlessly. Lister believed that applying some simple sanitary techniques, as Semmelweis had done, might save some lives.

In 1864, at a hospital in Glasgow, Scotland, Lister began using carbolic acid as an antiseptic, or germ-killing agent. He applied a cloth soaked in the acid to wounds caused by serious bone fractures. Normally, nearly half the patients with these wounds died of a serious infection called gas gangrene. Lister tested the antiseptic for one year. By the end of the year, the death rate for fracture cases had dropped to 10 percent. This convinced Lister that germs did enter wounds through the air. So

Austrian doctor Ignaz Semmelweis asked doctors to wash their hands with a chlorine rinse before touching their patients.

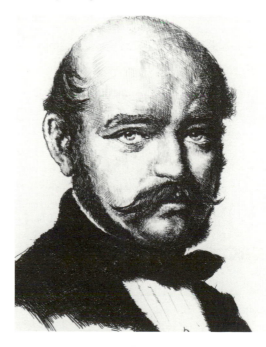

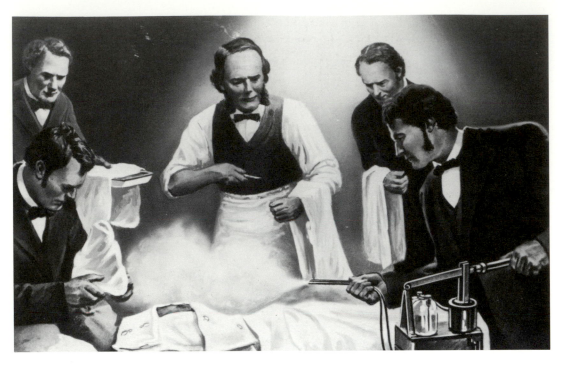

Lister believed germs entered open wounds through the air. Here, he sprays a germ-killing chemical into the air surrounding a patient.

he rigged a device that sprayed a germ-killing substance into the air in the hospital's operating rooms. In time, he learned that the risk of infection was far greater from germs on bed linens and human hands than from germs in the air. This prompted him to stop spraying and introduce strict rules about sterilizing hands, linens, and medical instruments to remove the germs on them.

Most doctors and hospitals were slow in adopting Lister's techniques. There was still a great deal of skepticism about the germ theory in the medical community. But Lister's work had an important effect on the progress of the germ theory. The results of Lister's experiments lent strong support to Pasteur and the other scientists who labored to prove the connection between germs and disease. Many researchers believed that Lister's success with antiseptics was valuable, indirect evidence that the germ theory was correct.

The Germ Theory Proven at Last

One researcher who closely followed the work of Pasteur, Virchow, Lister, and others was the German scientist Robert Koch. Like the others, Koch was convinced that germs cause disease. He hoped to prove the connection between the two by studying anthrax, a fatal disease that struck cattle, sheep, and other domesticated animals.

Koch had one important advantage over other researchers. One of the problems early microbiologists regularly encountered was that most germs did not live very long on a microscope slide. Without constant warmth, the germs died before scientists could observe their complete life cycle under magnification. Koch designed and built a special "warm-stage" microscope that allowed him to keep anthrax bacteria alive for much longer periods of time. With this invention, he could view almost the whole reproductive cycle under his microscope.

Koch knew that periodic epidemics of anthrax wiped out herds of sheep and cattle throughout Europe. He suspected that germs infected and killed the animals, then entered the soil. Somehow, the germs managed to stay alive in the soil, Koch reasoned. Later, healthy animals became infected when they came into contact with the germs in the soil. Koch believed that this was why the disease remained dormant, or inactive, for a while and then later reappeared.

In his laboratory, Koch injected mice and other animals with the blood of sheep that had recently died of anthrax. He found that all of the animals injected contracted the disease. He also

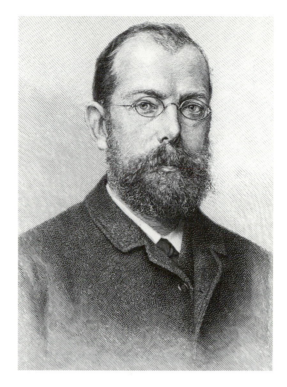

German scientist Robert Koch used a "warm-stage" microscope to study anthrax, a disease fatal to sheep, cattle, and domestic animals.

saw that all the dead animals had a certain kind of rod-shaped bacteria in their blood. Koch believed these were the

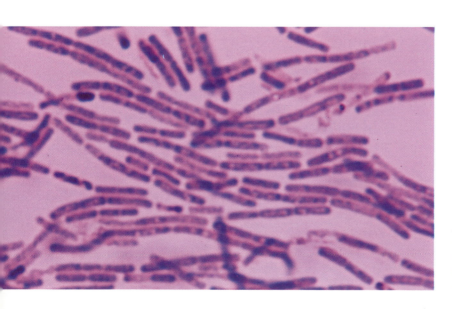

Anthrax bacteria, seen here, eventually change into tiny spores that transmit anthrax to animals.

BACTERIA FORMS CHAINS

SPORES THAT FORM IN LATER STAGES

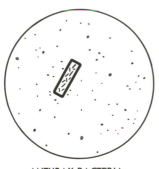

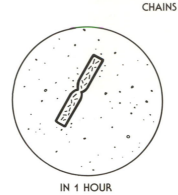

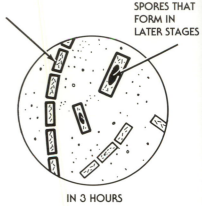

ANTHRAX BACTERIA

IN 1 HOUR

IN 3 HOURS

Anthrax is a disease that infects cattle, sheep, and other warm-blooded animals and can be transmitted to people.

Anthrax bacteria reproduce by dividing. In one hour, the bacteria split in two. In three hours, the bacteria split several times to form a chain. Eventually, the chain transforms into tiny seedlike particles known as spores. People and animals may become infected with anthrax when they come into contact with soil, hair, or other products that are infected with anthrax spores.

bacteria that caused the disease. He placed some of the bacteria under his warm-stage microscope and watched them grow. After several hours, the rods changed, forming a complex tangle of threads. The threads eventually transformed into tiny spores, or seedlike particles. Koch now needed to answer two questions. First, were these spores a reproductive stage of the disease? Second, could they infect healthy animals? If the spores did cause the animals to contract anthrax, it would mean that the spores were what transmitted the disease.

Koch injected some of the spores into lab mice. The mice soon came down with anthrax. He observed the blood of the mice under his microscope. Instead of spores, there were millions of the rod-shaped bacteria, identical to the ones that he had started with. This proved that the bacteria reproduced through spores.

The way the anthrax disease cycle worked was now clear to Koch. Bacteria in diseased animals changed into spores, and some of these spores entered the soil. Tough and resistant to temperature extremes, the spores remained in the soil for months or years. The disease would lie dormant until a healthy animal came along and ingested the spores by eating food grown in the soil. Once in the animal's warm blood, the spores reproduced and the disease spread.

In 1876, Koch presented his findings to German scientists at the University of Breslau. From there, the news traveled all over the world that Koch had established the connection between germs and disease. The germ theory became almost universally ac-

ease of animals and that Koch had shown only that germs could infect and kill animals. They insisted there still was no proof that germs cause human diseases. Koch, Pasteur, and their colleagues, confident that the germ theory was well-established, ignored these criticisms. The few remaining doubters were silenced in 1882, when Koch discovered the bacteria that caused tuberculosis. This discovery proved that germs not only cause disease in animals but also in people.

Countless Shapes and Behaviors

Scientists realized that by confirming the germ theory, they had taken only a tiny step toward understanding the problem of disease. For one thing, there were many different kinds of germs, and researchers knew very little about their various behaviors. In Koch and Pasteur's time, scientists recognized four general categories of germs: bacteria, fungi, protozoa, and algae. There were tens of thousands of different

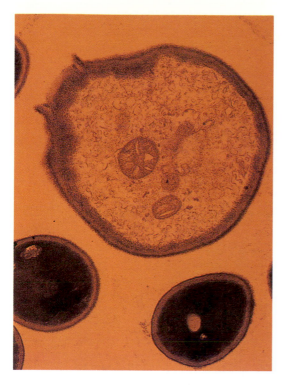

Yeasts are a type of microscopic fungus. Yeasts played an important role in Pasteur's initial experiments with wine and fermentation. Here, a yeast cell is seen magnified forty thousand times.

cepted by scientists. Incredibly, a few researchers still refused to accept the theory. They argued that anthrax was a dis-

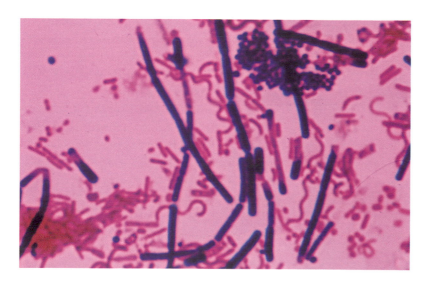

Bacteria, as seen through an electron microscope, come in different shapes and sizes. These include rods, spirals, and spheres.

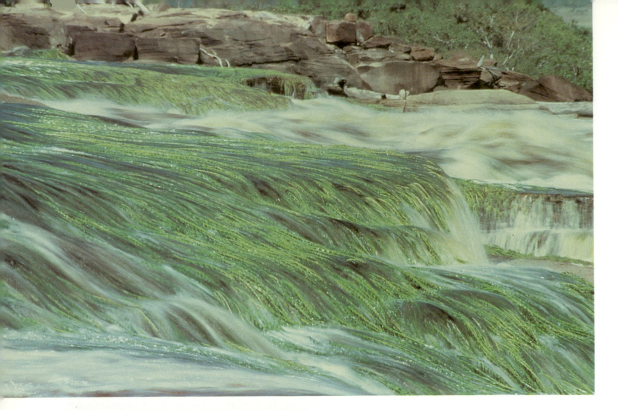

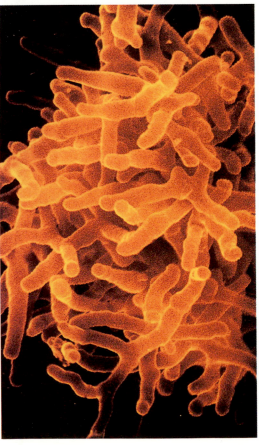

(top) Algae , a type of germ, are found predominantly in water. Algae contain chlorophyll which produces oxygen during photosynthesis. Algae are also the first living link on the food chain. (bottom) Threadlike bacteria magnified fourteen thousand times.

types of germs in each category. Over the course of several decades, researchers proved the existence of a fifth category—viruses—and learned much more about germs. Microbiologists found that germs exhibit thousands of different shapes and behaviors. Most often, they are single-celled organisms that multiply very rapidly.

Bacteria are relatively simple and reproduce by dividing in half, a process called fission. They can live in a wide variety of environments and temperatures. Some bacteria need oxygen to survive, while others live without oxygen. Some bacteria cause diseases, such as cholera, but many others are harmless and live in and actually benefit the bodies of animals and people.

KINDS OF GERMS

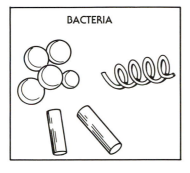

BACTERIA

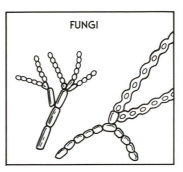

FUNGI

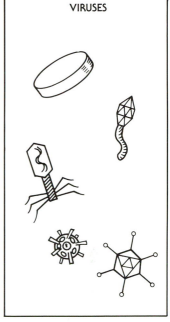

VIRUSES

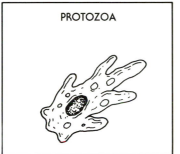

PROTOZOA

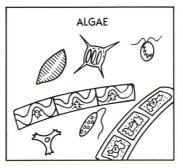

ALGAE

There are thousands of types of germs. Scientists recognize five general kinds of germs: bacteria, fungi, protozoa, algae, and viruses.

Bacteria are typically spherical, rodlike, or spirallike. Fungi sometimes resemble a chain or string of beads.

Protozoa take many different configurations ranging from shapeless blobs to symmetrical forms. Algae can be spherical, rectangular, or irregular in shape. Viruses are corkscrew-shaped strands that are much smaller than other kinds of germs.

Some fungi, such as mushrooms, are not germs. It is the microscopic variety of fungi, including the single-celled yeasts, that are referred to as germs. Yeasts are oval-shaped and are much larger than bacteria. When yeasts come in contact with certain substances, they cause the process of fermentation to occur. They also cause the decay of dead plant and animal tissue. Some fungal germs reproduce by releasing spores, which spread by wind and water.

Protozoa are large germs with rela-

tively complex internal structures. They reproduce when their nuclei, or central sections, divide. This process is called mitosis. Protozoa live in water and other liquids. They move almost constantly, propelled by tiny pseudopods, or false feet. Protozoa often live in the bodies of animals or humans and can cause such diseases as malaria and sleeping sickness.

Algae come in many shapes and sizes. The most common forms, called diatoms, float in vast numbers in the oceans. These contain a green substance

(right) The Epstein-Barr virus, discovered in 1968, causes mononucleosis and is associated with other diseases. (below) A scientist observes germs through an electron microscope. These microscopes use beams of electrons, rather than light, to magnify extremely small objects.

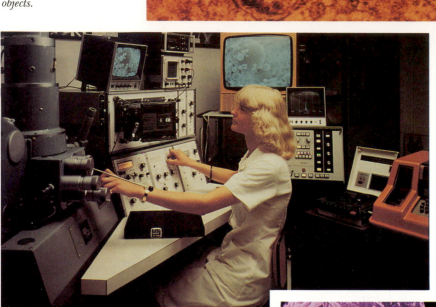

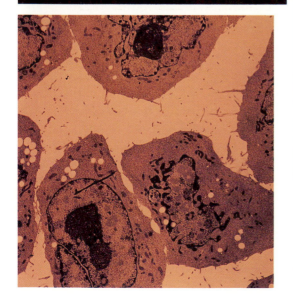

These human body cells (left) are infected with adenovirus, a type of virus that causes respiratory diseases and induces malignant tumors. (above) A human immunodeficiency virus (HIV) emerges from a human blood cell.

HOW THE INFLUENZA VIRUS INVADES A CELL

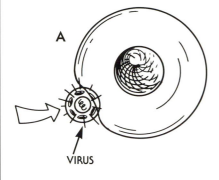

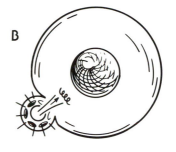

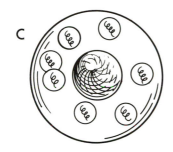

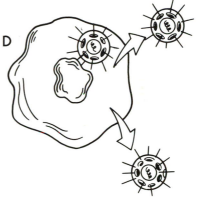

VIRUS

When the influenza virus invades the body, the virus attaches itself to a healthy cell (A). It then breaks through the cell wall (B). Once inside the healthy cell, the virus multiplies and the once-healthy cell dies (C). The newly formed virus particles escape and attack other cells and the process begins again.

called chlorophyll, which the algae use in a process called photosynthesis. In this process, sunlight and carbon dioxide from the air combine in the presence of chlorophyll to form "food" for the algae. The process releases oxygen as a by-product. Most of the oxygen in the earth's atmosphere is produced in this manner by ocean algae. Algae are also a food source for larger organisms, such as fish, and form the base of nature's food chain. Most algae do not cause disease.

Viruses are very different from the other types of germs. Viruses are hun-dreds and sometimes thousands of times smaller than the others. In fact, viruses are so tiny that they can be seen only with specialized, very powerful microscopes. These organisms are not true cells, as bacteria and other types of germs are. Viruses are tiny, corkscrew-shaped strands made up of two simple materials, nucleic acid and protein. Viruses can reproduce only inside the living cells of other organisms. Because of this dependence on other organisms, viruses are considered parasites. While living within these cells, viruses often cause serious diseases, such as smallpox and rabies.

Like the other kinds of germs, viruses cause disease by attacking the cells of the host—the plant, animal, or person the germs have invaded. Some germs bore into the cells, damaging them. Others partially digest the cells. Most germs also give off poisons, called toxins, which not only destroy the cells but also travel through the host's bloodstream. The toxins often produce serious physical side effects, such as fever, heart problems, and diarrhea.

Because there are so many different kinds of germs, work was slow and difficult for the early scientists who searched for ways to conquer disease. The researchers found that some diseases affected plants only, while others, like anthrax, killed animals. Some dis-eases, like bubonic plague, killed both animals and people. One of the most significant discoveries was that not all diseases spread the same way. The distribution of spores, as in anthrax, was only one of many ways.

So, the late 1800s and early 1900s became a period of intensive research in the new field of microbiology. It was painstaking, often frustrating work. Scientists had to tackle each disease separately. First, they had to find out which germ was involved, then explain the way it attacked the host, and finally, determine how the disease spread. More than two hundred years had passed since van Leeuwenhoek first observed germs, yet science had only just begun to discover the secrets of nature's smallest creatures.

Tracking the Spread of Disease Germs

The work of Pasteur, Virchow, Koch, and others firmly established that germs cause disease. This knowledge made it easier to track the spread of disease because now, at least, scientists knew what to look for even if they did not know exactly where to look. Nevertheless, many challenges lay ahead. More powerful microscopes came into use in the late 1800s, allowing researchers to study germs in increasingly greater detail. Experiments involving germs were conducted in labs in Germany, Great Britain, the United States, Italy, France, and other countries.

The ultimate goal of scientists and doctors was to find effective cures for the various diseases. But these researchers knew that goal would be difficult and would take time to achieve. Finding out how each disease attacked

the body would be a slow process.

The scientists also realized that finding cures for diseases was not the only way to save lives. If people knew how a particular disease spread, the germs that caused that disease might be controlled. Once Robert Koch revealed that anthrax spores lay dormant in the

Pasteur, Virchow, Koch, and other scientists had no access to powerful microscopes. Today's electron microscope can magnify objects up to a million times.

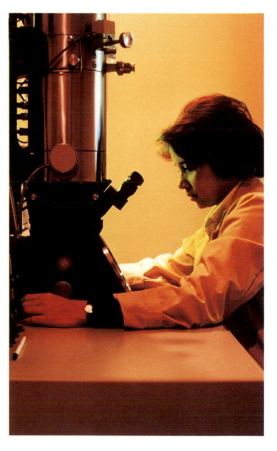

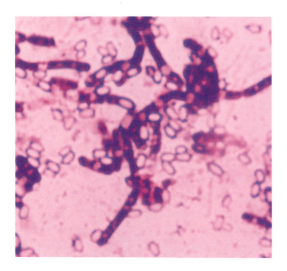

Bacillus spores, as seen through a microscope.

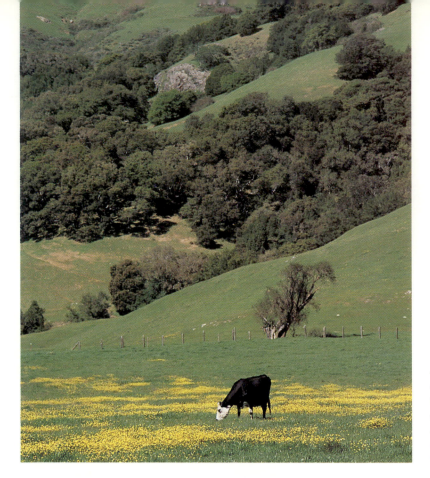

Anthrax spores can lie dormant in soil. For this reason, scientists test soil samples for the deadly disease before allowing cattle and other animals to graze.

soil, for example, scientists could easily determine if the spores were present by testing samples of soil from various fields. Cattle could then be moved to spore-free fields where they would be safe from the disease even if no treatment for anthrax were available.

Tracking the spread of disease was the first step in learning how to control that disease. This is why some of the most important studies about germs and disease in the early days of microbiology took place in outside laboratories. Some researchers went into the "field," which meant that they traveled from town to town, or country to country, searching for clues about how germs infected people. Not surprisingly, these researchers paid the most attention to those diseases that were the most deadly. Certain killer plagues, for example, repeatedly struck large populations. Learning to control these diseases would eliminate much death and suffering.

Mass Death in Africa

For many centuries, one of the worst epidemic, or rapidly spreading, diseases was sleeping sickness, which repeatedly wiped out entire villages and tribes in many sections of Africa. The symptoms of sleeping sickness were unmistakable and devastating. In the first stage of the illness, the victim had constant headaches and felt tired and depressed. The person also suffered from insomnia, the inability to sleep. This stage of sleeping sickness often lasted for several months or even a few years. During this time, the victim was unable to function normally and became a burden on both family and community, which often made the person feel useless and even more depressed. In the second stage of the disease, the victim lost the ability to reason and think clearly. Severe pains racked most of the body, and the person was constantly drowsy, usually sleeping away much of the day as well as the night. Eventually, the victim lapsed into a coma and, in nearly all cases, died.

Sleeping sickness, called *Lumbe* in some parts of Central Africa, spread to the Central African nation of Uganda in the late 1800s. This was a densely populated area, and the disease caused widespread suffering and death. Between 1900 and 1907, nearly 200,000 people died from sleeping sickness in Uganda. The British, who had controlled the country since 1894, were alarmed. British medical personnel worried not only about the huge loss of life in Uganda but also about the possibility

that the disease might spread to Egypt and to other areas, killing thousands more.

Solving the Mystery of Sleeping Sickness

The British sent an official Sleeping Sickness Commission to Uganda in 1902. Members of the commission tried to find out how the disease spread by mapping the outbreaks in specific villages. They found a definite pattern of infection. The disease occurred only on lake islands or in villages located on lakeshores and along riverbanks. There were no important outbreaks of the sickness in areas far from water. Some of the commission doctors reasoned that there must be dangerous germs in the water and that people caught the disease by drinking contaminated water. This explanation seemed logical, based

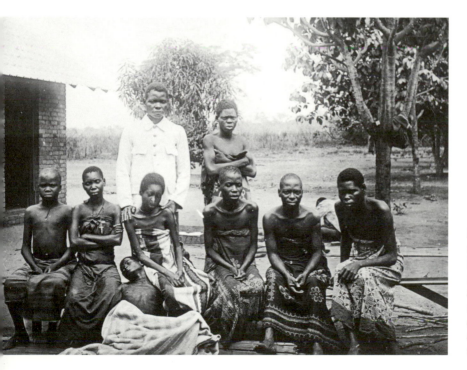

Sleeping sickness spread to the African nation of Uganda in the late 1800s and continues to afflict people in some countries. Here, victims of the disease show signs of drowsiness and weight loss.

DISEASE-CAUSING BACTERIA

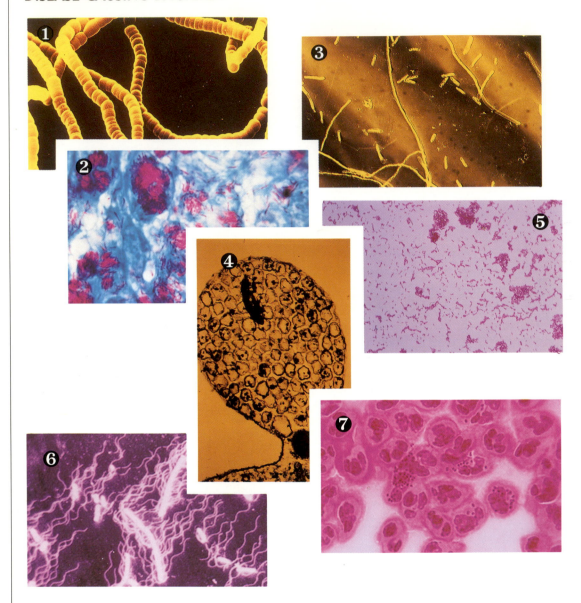

These bacteria have at least one thing in common—they all cause disease. *Streptococcus bacterium* (1) causes sore throats. *Mycobacterium leprae* (2) causes leprosy. *Legionella* (3) causes Legionnaire's disease. *Rickettsia* (4) causes typhus. *Shigella dysenterioe* (5) causes dysentery, a disease characterized by severe diarrhea. *Salmonella typhosa* (6) causes typhoid fever. *Neisterio gonorrhoeae* (7) causes gonorrhea.

on the experiences of one British doctor nearly fifty years earlier in London. That doctor, named John Snow, did not know what caused disease, but through painstaking investigation, he discovered the source of the city's recurrent cholera epidemics was to be found in a city drinking water pump.

Doctors with the Sleeping Sickness Commission followed Snow's example and initally concluded that contaminated drinking water was also the cause of Uganda's epidemic. But, unlike Snow, the commission doctors were able to test the water for the presence of disease germs. What they found was puzzling. Initial examination of the local water found no potentially harmful germs.

In 1903, a second commission arrived in Uganda to study sleeping sickness. The team of researchers was led by Dr. David Bruce, an army medical officer. Bruce looked at the findings of the first commission and offered a different theory of how the disease spread. According to Bruce, the doctors found no harmful germs in the water because the disease did not spread through the water itself.

Infected Tsetse Flies

Bruce had recently studied a disease that killed livestock in northern Africa. He had succeeded in isolating the germ that caused the disease, showing that it was a protozoan that infected tsetse flies, large relatives of ordinary houseflies. When the flies bit an animal, the protozoa entered the animal's bloodstream and contaminated it. Bruce suggested that sleeping sickness might be spreading among humans in the same manner.

Bruce ordered a study of the distribution of tsetse flies in the area. The researchers found that the flies bred by laying their eggs in water. They also found that the areas where the flies bred and lived were exactly the same areas where outbreaks of sleeping sickness occurred. Bruce examined the flies and found a protozoan parasite called *Trypanosoma*. He exposed laboratory monkeys to tsetse flies infected with this parasite. All of the test animals developed sleeping sickness. Another piece of evidence emerged when one of Bruce's colleagues, Dr. Aldo Castellani, found trypanosomes in the spinal fluid of human sleeping sickness victims.

Bruce and his team proved that sleeping sickness affected human populations living near water because the

During the influenza outbreak of 1918, this poster warned people about the dangers of infecting others.

INFLUENZA
FREQUENTLY COMPLICATED WITH
PNEUMONIA
IS PREVALENT AT THIS TIME THROUGHOUT AMERICA.
THIS THEATRE IS CO-OPERATING WITH THE DEPARTMENT OF HEALTH.
YOU MUST DO THE SAME
IF YOU HAVE A COLD AND ARE COUGHING AND SNEEZING DO NOT ENTER THIS THEATRE
GO HOME AND GO TO BED UNTIL YOU ARE WELL

Coughing, Sneezing or Spitting Will Not Be Permitted In The Theatre. In case you must cough or Sneeze, do so in your own handkerchief, and if the Coughing or Sneezing Persists Leave The Theatre At Once.

This Theatre has agreed to co-operate with the Department Of Health in disseminating the truth about Influenza, and thus serve a great educational purpose.

HELP US TO KEEP CHICAGO THE HEALTHIEST CITY IN THE WORLD
JOHN DILL ROBERTSON
COMMISSIONER OF HEALTH

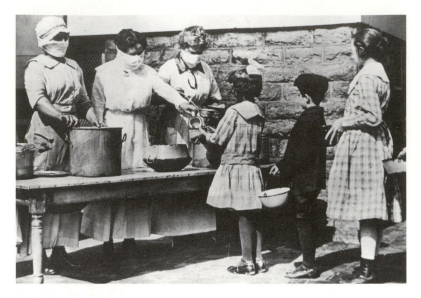

In 1917, influenza afflicted millions of people. Here, volunteers in Cincinnati wear protective gauze masks while they feed children of families stricken with the virus.

flies that carried the disease germs could only breed in water. There was still no cure for the disease but understanding how it spread offered hope that sleeping sickness might be controlled. In 1907, Hesketh Bell, the British administrator in charge of Uganda, convinced the local chiefs to move their villages away from lakes and rivers. This relocation resulted in a dramatic reduction in the incidence of sleeping sickness. Unfortunately, infected tsetse flies remained. Despite repeated efforts to wipe out the insects during the twentieth century, the flies continued to spread the disease in isolated areas. Although the disease no longer wipes out whole villages, deaths from sleeping sickness in Africa have been reported as recently as 1990.

The Disease Detectives

Bruce and his colleagues took the knowledge that germs cause disease into the field and showed one of the many ways that diseases are transmitted.

They and other researchers helped establish some of the basic guidelines and foundations of the science of epidemiology, the systematic study of disease epidemics. Epidemiologists are, in a sense, disease detectives who track down

This woman wears a flu mask during the 1919 influenza outbreak.

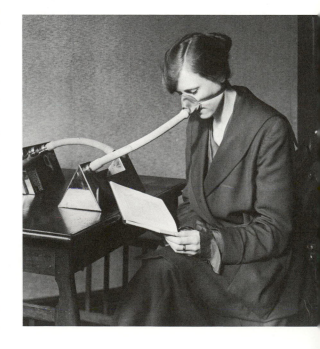

clues to the various ways germs spread disease.

Epidemiologists learned from the beginning that explaining how a particular disease spread did not mean the disease had been beaten, even when a cure was known. New outbreaks of a disease could occur at any time and spread in different ways. What made the job of the epidemiologist easier, was knowing exactly what kind of germ to look for. Not knowing sometimes sent them down the wrong trails.

Such was the case with influenza, more commonly known as flu. For many years, doctors had a difficult time determining how influenza spread. From their research, they knew it did not spread through insects. Nor was it transmitted to humans by spores or bacteria that grow in unsanitary conditions.

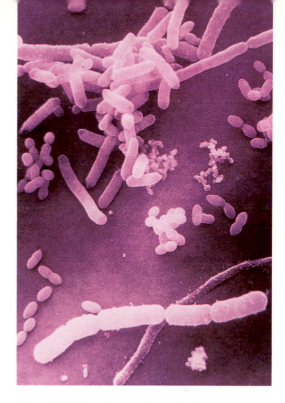

Bacteria inside a human intestinal tract, as seen through an electron microscope.

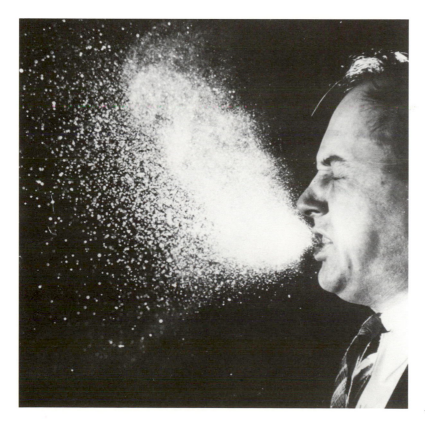

When a person sneezes, droplets from the mouth and nose spread at a rate of up to 150 feet per second. When most of the droplets evaporate, thousands of germ-carrying particles are left floating in the air.

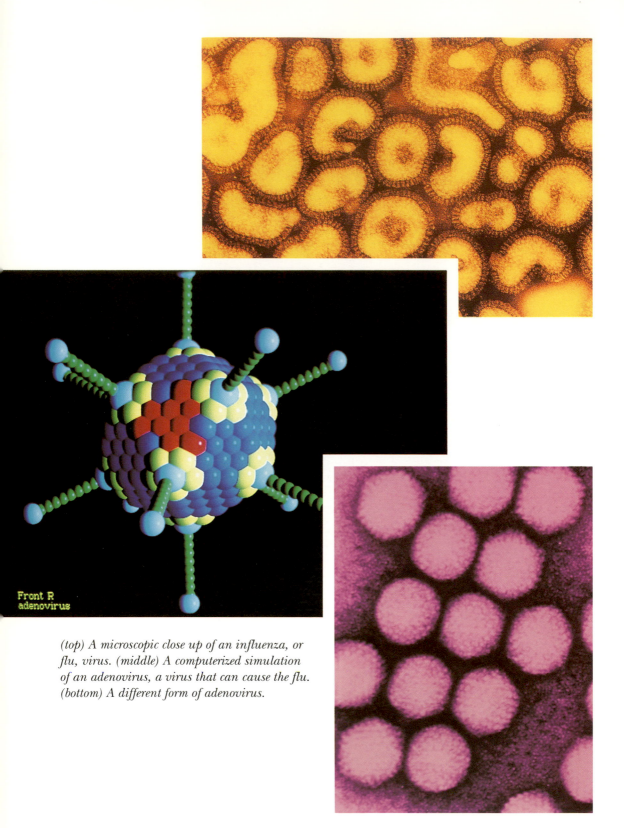

(top) A microscopic close up of an influenza, or flu, virus. (middle) A computerized simulation of an adenovirus, a virus that can cause the flu. (bottom) A different form of adenovirus.

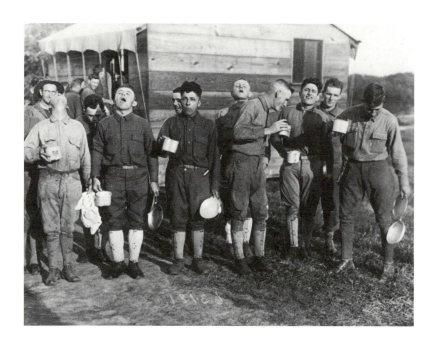

In 1917, military men gargle with salt and hot water to protect themselves against influenza.

What doctors did know all too well was that influenza could be deadly. Between 1918 and 1919, influenza killed at least 20 million people worldwide. In the United States alone, more than 550,000 people, or ten times the number of Americans killed in World War I, died of influenza. The epidemic was so bad that medical officials opened an emergency hospital in Washington, D.C. Dr. James Leake, the head of the facility, said, "The only way we could find room for the sick was to have undertakers waiting at the door. . . . The living came in one door and the dead went out the other."

Looking for Clues

Efforts at identifying how influenza spread were complicated by the fact that its cause was unknown. Researchers could not see any germs in the body fluids of influenza victims. Nevertheless, the scientists mistakenly assumed that bacteria were the culprits and that they were just too small to see. Based on this assumption, doctors tried tracking and treating the disease with methods that had worked with other bacterial illnesses. But none of these methods worked. The disease did not appear to be caused by fungal or protozoal germs either. It was not until 1933 that scientists discovered that influenza was caused by an altogether different germ called a virus.

The invention of special, extremely powerful microscopes made this discovery possible. With these microscopes, researchers could detect viruses in body fluids for the first time. Many of these viruses were hundreds of times smaller than other germs. Because researchers found vast numbers of viruses in body fluids like mucus and saliva, they concluded that influenza passed from one person to another through the air. When a person coughs, sneezes, or even exhales, droplets of saliva and mucus loaded with viruses spray into the air.

VIRUSES

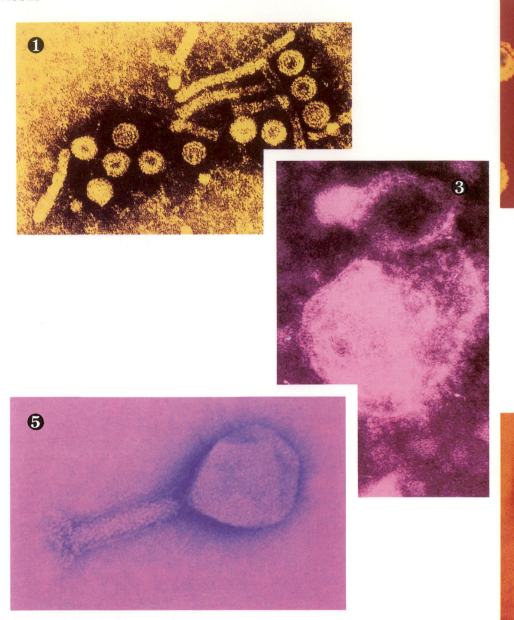

Viruses can be many sizes, shapes, and colors. They cause various diseases in plants and animals and can even attack bacteria. Shown here are magnified views of six viruses. Hepatitis (1), a disease that causes inflammation of the liver. Herpes, measles, and pox (2, 3, 4), which are characterized by eruptions on the skin. Bacteriophage (5), a virus that eats various types of bacteria. Rabies (6), a disease that afflicts the nervous system of mammals.

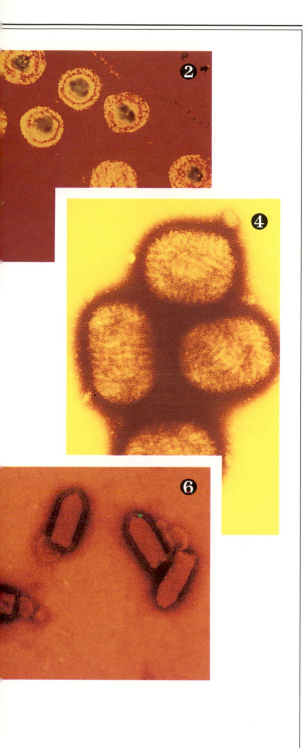

Other people breathe in the droplets, and the viruses enter the bloodstream through the air sacs in the lungs. Disease detectives found that influenza viruses can also pass from people into pigs, ducks, and other animals. The animals can carry the disease and then transmit it back to humans in similar ways.

Although they had discovered what causes influenza, researchers found that tracking the disease was still difficult. The influenza virus seemed capable of changing its form. Sometimes, epidemiologists were not sure if they were dealing with one disease or many similar diseases. Eventually, they learned that viruses can mutate, or change, easily,

The DNA strands can be seen in this virus that is magnified forty-eight thousand times.

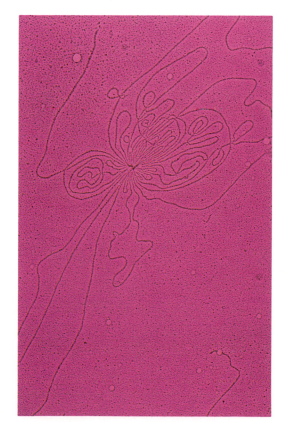

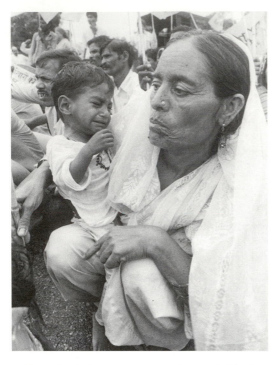

forming new strains of diseases. A new strain of a disease may be resistant to medicines that were effective against a former strain. This has been the case with influenza. It keeps returning, and each time, medical experts must develop new medicines to combat it. They also must be on the alert for the possibility that a mutated form of the disease might begin spreading in a completely different way. Researchers still worry about this possibility. Alan Kendal of the Centers for Disease Control in Atlanta, Georgia, says, "Believe me, we have every reason to be afraid of this virus. Every year it claims thousands of lives in the U.S. When a new strain appears, hundreds of thousands of people may die around the world." Kendal admits that scientists still know relatively little about flu viruses. "We don't know what made [the 1918 outbreak] so deadly. And there is always the chance that another one will strike," he said.

(above) An Indian woman comforts a child who is suffering from cholera. Cholera can cause severe diarrhea and vomiting. (below left) A magnified view of cholera bacteria found in the intestinal lining. (below right) The cholera bacteria.

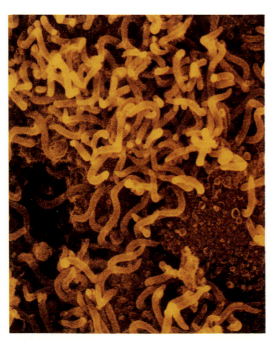

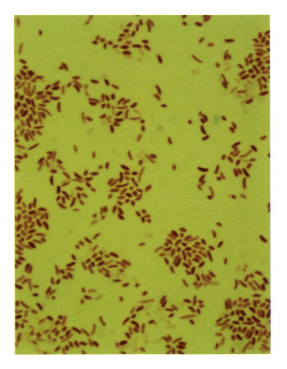

Sticking to Basics

Although knowledge about germs and disease has greatly increased during the twentieth century, today's disease detectives use many of the same basic methods their predecessors used. The primary tool of epidemiology is still fieldwork. In this tradition, epidemiologist Nathan Shaffer set out in 1987 to help doctors in the small African nation of Guinea-Bissau stop a massive outbreak of cholera. Since the days of John Snow, cholera has continued to plague humanity. Serious cholera epidemics swept large areas of the world in 1899 and 1923 and then again in the 1970s. In 1978 alone, seventy-five thousand people worldwide died of cholera.

With this in mind, Shaffer immediately began his detective work. He had to figure out how the disease was infecting people, both on the seacoast and in the inland areas. He knew that cholera often spread through contaminated water. "But," explained Shaffer, "the outbreaks didn't seem to be associated with particular wells. . . . The epidemic was spreading up and down the coast. Right away, I suspected shellfish."

He thought of shellfish because he knew they often carry water-borne diseases. Shaffer went from house to house, asking people how and when they became ill and what they ate. And he asked questions about everyday hygiene. He tested shellfish from local markets and found cholera bacteria. This explained how the people on the coast had contracted the disease. But eighty people had died from cholera in an inland village. Shaffer traveled to the village and found that none of the victims had eaten shellfish from the coast.

Shaffer searched for clues to the mystery. He learned that one of the villagers was a dockworker on the coast. He had recently died of cholera, and his body had been shipped home. Shaffer then discovered that some of the

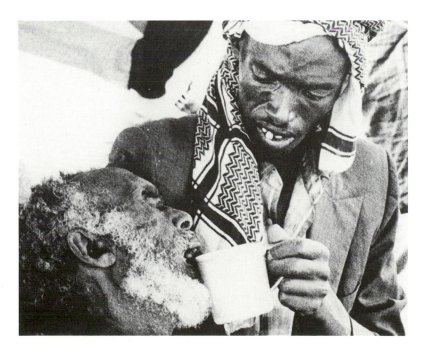

One symptom of cholera is severe dehydration. Here, a man offers rehydration salts to his elderly father who is suffering from the disease.

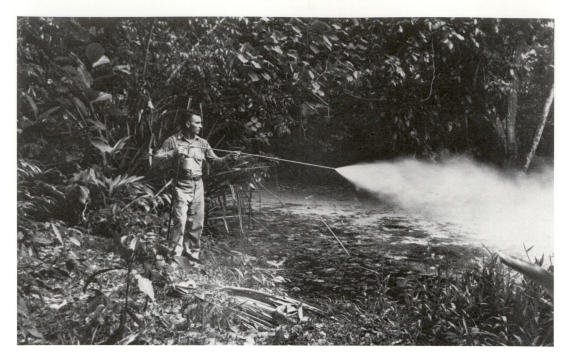

Scientists have known for many years that insects may carry disease. During World War II, mosquitos infected troops stationed in the Pacific with malaria and other diseases. Here, a marine in Guadalcanal sprays insecticides to kill mosquitos.

same people who handled the body during the burial also helped prepare the funeral feast. Investigating further, Shaffer found that more than half of the people who attended the feast contracted cholera.

Disease detectives like Shaffer realize that they must always be prepared to fight new outbreaks of diseases such as cholera. In 1991, in fact, Peru and other South American nations were fighting a new and dangerous cholera epidemic. As one writer said of the disease, "It remains hovering in the wings like a sinister shadow, ever patient, awaiting its chance once again to carry death abroad in the world."

Scientists and doctors realize that diseases like sleeping sickness, cholera, and influenza will affect humanity for a long time to come. They say that one important way to combat the germs that cause these plagues is to control their spread. Methods might include destroying disease-carrying insects, instituting better sanitation methods, being more careful about eating certain foods, and isolating infected individuals from others. And, modern disease detectives must continue to identify the ways in which germs move through the environment and infect plants and animals. Someday, human beings may win the war against dangerous germs. Until that day comes, people must continue to fight and win one battle at a time.

Identifying Useful Germs

Not all germs are dangerous and destructive. During the golden age of microbiology, while scientists studied harmful germs, it became clear that many germs are harmless. In fact, researchers discovered that only a small fraction of the germs that exist in nature cause disease. The vast majority are actually beneficial to plants, animals, and humans. Scientists have established that without germs, these higher forms of life could not exist.

Just as Pasteur suggested, germs exist almost everywhere in the environment. In countless numbers, they float through the air on dust particles and swim through the oceans. They live in the soil and in sewage. Germs have been found in such inhospitable places as frozen Antarctic wastelands and boiling hot springs.

Germs Work in the Environment

Most of these germs have become part of the planet's natural cycles. Germs are involved in the processes that nurture life as well as the processes of decay, which make room for new growth. For example, certain types of germs in the soil help plants consume nitrogen from the air. Without nitrogen, plants cannot live, and without plants, many animals cannot live. Because people eat both an-

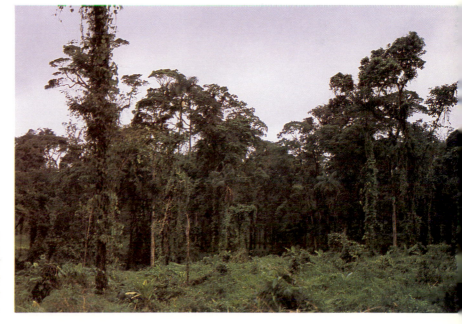

Certain types of germs are actually beneficial to plants. Germs in the soil help plants consume useful nutrients from the air.

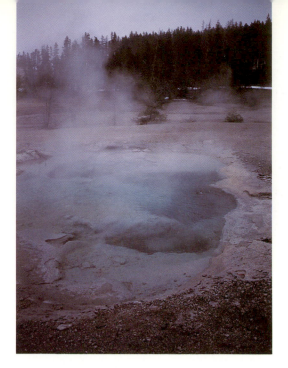

Germs live everywhere. They are found in every environment from frozen Antarctic wastelands to boiling hot springs

synthesis, ocean algae take in carbon dioxide and give off oxygen. Algae are also important because they form the basis of nature's food chain. Tiny animals eat the algae and then are themselves eaten by larger animals. Eventually, humans eat some of these animals. In this way, humans indirectly depend on the algae for food.

Other types of germs live by consuming the tissue of dead plants and animals. In this process, germs release chemicals that cause dead things to decay. As the dead tissues are broken down into simpler substances, these compounds are recycled back into the environment for use by living plants and animals. As germs break down dead tissues, for example, they release elements such as carbon, nitrogen, and phosphorus into the air and soil. Plants take in these elements and use them to build their own tissues. Animals then consume the plants. When these living things die, the process repeats itself. These are only some of the ways in which germs help sustain the earth's

imals and plants, they also depend on the germs that help plants take nitrogen from the air.

Germs also help supply most of the oxygen that animals and humans need to live. Through the process of photo-

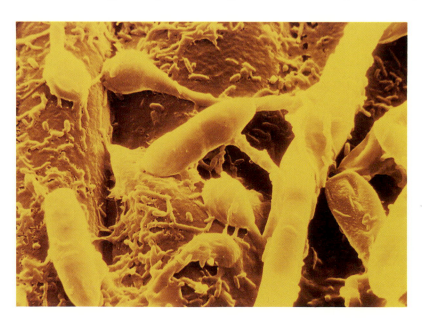

Germs are important to life and nature. Germs cause dead things to decay, providing nutrients for new life. Here, a microscopic view of fungi and bacteria on a root surface.

GERMS' ROLE IN NATURE'S FOOD CHAIN

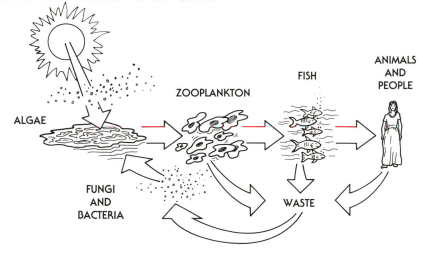

The food chain begins in the ocean, where microscopic plants such as algae consume sunlight and carbon dioxide from the air and nutrients from the water. Tiny animals such as zooplankton then eat the algae. These tiny animals become food for larger animals such as fish. Humans and other animals eat the fish.

The waste products of all these creatures are broken down by germs such as fungi and bacteria. These broken-down wastes become food for other creatures and the cycle begins again.

natural cycles. Pasteur recognized the importance of these germs when he said, "Life would not long remain possible in the absence of microbes."

At Home on People

With so many germs in the air, soil, and water, it is not surprising that germs exist on people, too. At any given moment, a clean, healthy person has literally trillions of harmless germs on both the inside and outside of the body. Microbiologists estimate that there are about thirty million germs on an area of human skin the size of a postage stamp. There are even more germs inside the body. There, more than one billion may exist in a space the size of a kernel of corn.

Unlike disease germs, which attack the body's cells and tissues, these germs live in and on the body and help keep it running properly. The harmless varieties live in cavities such as the mouth and rectum, in the intestines, and in open spaces between the organs. Most of these tiny creatures take advantage of the warmth, moisture, and nutrients available in the body. They live by consuming mucus, dead cells cast off by body parts, and various waste products. These germs have become very specialized, with specific kinds living only in specific areas of the body. Some types are so specialized that they cannot grow and thrive anywhere else in nature but

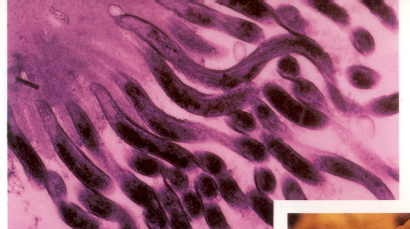

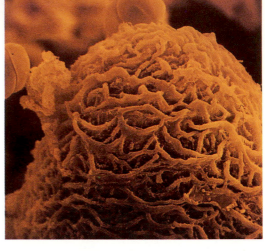

Some germs are so specialized that they can live only in certain parts of the human body. (left) Spiral-shaped bacteria in the intestinal tract. (below) Bacteria as seen on the edge of a fingerprint.

in a human body. Research indicates that just as some germs cannot live without people, people cannot live without some germs.

One way that germs help the body function properly is by stimulating the immune system. The purpose of the immune system is to fight infection and disease. All animals, including humans, have special cells that produce substances called antibodies. These are like tiny soldiers that attack and destroy harmful germs that penetrate the body's tissues. In a way that scientists still do not understand, useful germs stimulate the body to produce sufficient antibodies. The body relies on its good germs to help it defeat the bad germs.

By conducting experiments with animals specially raised in germ-free environments, scientists have shown that good germs stimulate the immune sys-

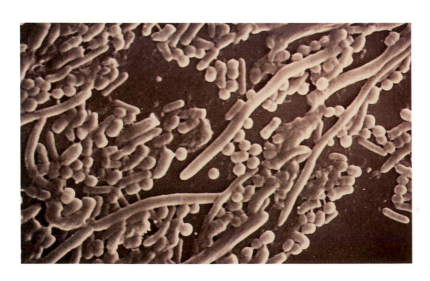

A close up view of the bacteria in dental plaque.

tem. These animals were never exposed to either good germs or harmful ones, and their immune systems did not function properly. The cells that make antibodies did not develop normally and, therefore, produced few antibodies. As a result, the animals' tissues and organs were wide open to attack by harmful disease germs.

Other Helpful Germs in the Body

Some germs make it possible for animals and people to digest food properly. The germs do this by ensuring that the intestines develop normally. The intestines are the long, folded tubes located in the lower abdomen. After food is partially digested in the stomach, the food passes into the intestines. There, further digestion takes place, and the nutrients in the food pass into the bloodstream. To work efficiently, the walls of the intestines must be of a certain thickness. And the muscles on the insides of the tubes must be strong enough to contract and push the food along.

Scientists do not know exactly how germs ensure normal intestinal development, but several experiments have suggested that they do play an impor-

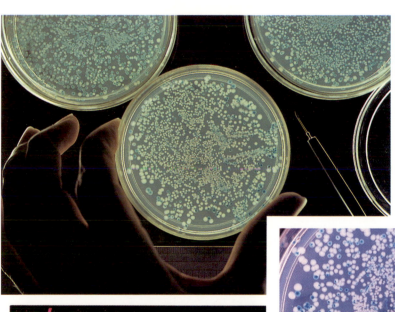

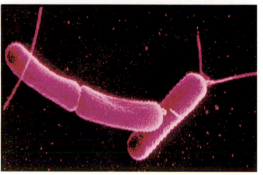

(left) Colonies of intestinal bacteria, called E. coli. (below left) E. coli bacteria as seen magnified thiry-five thousand times.(below right) A colony of E. coli bacteria infected with a bacteriophage, a type of virus that eats bacteria.

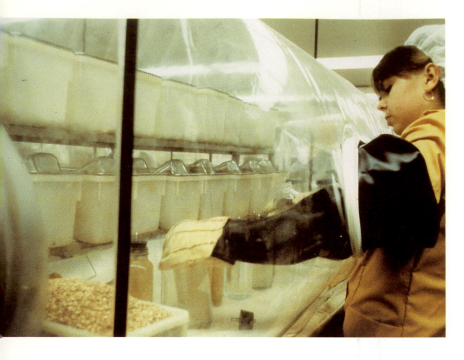

Scientists monitor an experimental germ-free environment to learn how the absence of germs affects plants and animals.

tant role. In these experiments, the researchers raised guinea pigs and other animals in completely germ-free environments. The intestines of these animals did not grow normally. The walls of the upper intestines were too thin, and the intestinal muscles were too weak to move the food along. Eventually, the animals died because their bodies could not absorb sufficient nutrients. Then, the researchers repeated the experiment, this time feeding intestinal bacteria to previously germ-free guinea pigs. Within a few weeks, the intestines of the animals grew thicker and stronger, and the guinea pigs digested their food normally. These experiments show that bacteria somehow induced the intestinal walls to grow to the proper thickness.

Germs also affect the way the heart pumps blood. The heart must pump a certain volume of blood each minute in order to keep fresh blood moving to the various parts of the body. The hearts of germ-free test animals pump a smaller volume of blood than the hearts of animals with normal germs. Scientists are not sure why or how this hap-

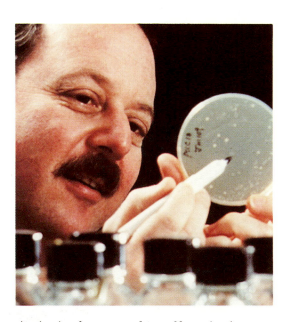

A scientist observes a culture of bacteria. A culture is a colony of bacteria grown in a laboratory.

HOW ANTIBODIES FIGHT THE INFLUENZA VIRUS

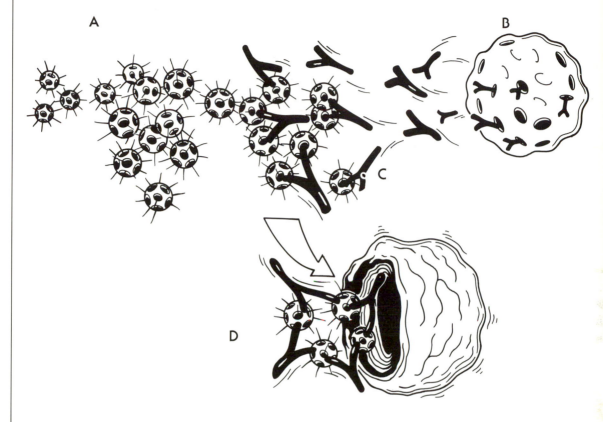

When the influenza virus invades the body (A), specialized cells produce antibodies (B). The antibodies seek out and attach themselves to the virus. The antibodies keep the virus from causing more damage to the body (C). Specialized "cleanup" cells digest the clustered antibodies and virus particles (D), leaving the body free from the harmful virus.

pens but confirm that the presence of germs in the body is essential to healthy blood circulation.

Germs also aid the body by producing many of the vitamins essential to good health. Certain germs in the intestines take in nutrients from food and chemically transform them into complex vitamins. Without these vitamins made by germs, people would be weak and unhealthy. The importance of these germs is revealed by what happens to people who are treated with drugs to stop infections. The drugs often kill large numbers of intestinal germs that normally make B vitamins. These vitamins are essential in breaking down important acids in the body as well as in the production of red blood cells, which carry oxygen throughout the body. Until the germ populations that make B vitamins are restored, these processes slow

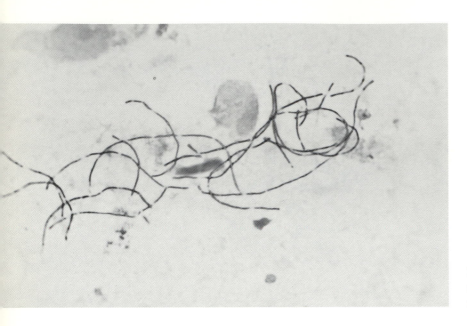

Lactobacillus is used in the production of many dairy products.

down, making the patients feel weak and uncomfortable.

All of these examples illustrate that useful germs and people enjoy a symbiosis, a relationship in which two living things benefit from living together. The fact that the human body does not develop or function properly without germs is significant. It suggests that as humans evolved and the body developed its form over the course of millions of years, germs evolved with them. This means that useful germs must have been present in the bodies of the most primitive ancestors of today's animals and people. Without germs, animals would not have evolved in the same way. Human beings, at least as we know them, might never have evolved at all.

Germs in Food Production

In addition to living in and on people, germs are also found in the foods people eat. Some of these germs harmlessly multiply on plant and animal products and later enter human digestive tracts. On the other hand, many important foods are actually produced with the aid of germs. This is another way that germs are beneficial to people.

A variety of dairy products are made with germs. These products take advantage of the fact that germs cause milk to spoil. Milk spoilage occurs when bacteria such as *Lactobacillus* attack the proteins, fats, and carbohydrates in milk. The milk sours and acquires a lumpy consistency called curd. When a carton of milk in the refrigerator sours, most people say the milk has gone bad and pour it down the drain. But certain kinds of milk spoilage—including curd—sometimes aid food production.

Buttermilk, for example, is made by adding cultures of bacteria to vats of pasteurized milk. A culture is a colony of bacteria grown in a laboratory. The bacteria cause the milk to ferment, just as yeast causes grape juice to ferment into wine. When the fermented milk is sour enough, it is ready to be packaged as buttermilk and shipped to stores. A

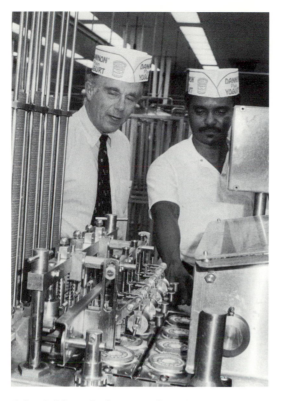

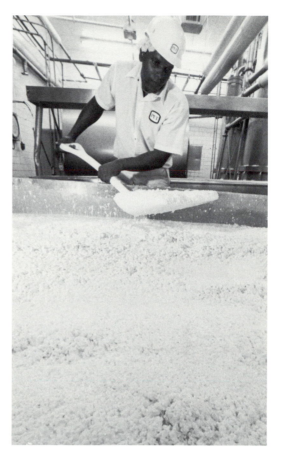

(above) Many foods are made with the help of germs, including yogurt. (above right) A worker at a dairy plant in Florida blends cream and cottage cheese.

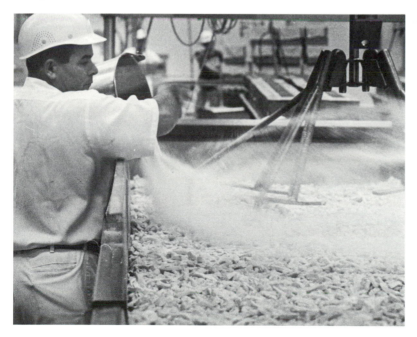

A dairy worker spreads salt on the curd of cheddar cheese.

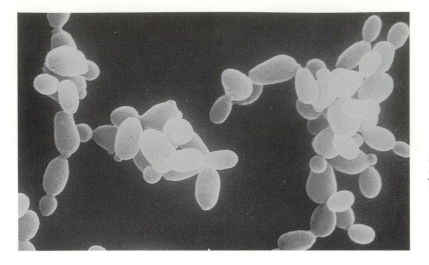

Special varieties of yeasts are used in baking, brewing, and winemaking. Here, budding yeasts are magnified thirteen thousand times.

few extra steps in the same process produce a thicker product popularly known as sour cream.

Yogurt is another dairy product made with germs. The first step in preparing yogurt is to boil milk until it becomes thick like custard. Next, cultures of *Lactobacillus* and other bacteria are added and the milk sours, just as it does when it gets old in the refrigerator. Finally, the product undergoes evaporation to remove some of the water content and thicken it further.

Perhaps the most important dairy product made with germs is cheese. The curd that forms when milk spoils is essentially an unripened form of cheese. Various forms of this curd are sold as cottage cheese, ricotta cheese, and cream cheese. Ripened cheeses, such as Swiss, Romano, and cheddar also use the curds of spoiled milk. The curds are pressed and salted. The salt adds taste and also keeps the curds from molding. Next, the curds are cut into the desired shape, and certain bacteria are added. The cheese is allowed to ripen for several months. During this time, the bac-

Yeasts cause grape juice to ferment and become wine. Here, a wine maker checks the sugar content in a new batch of wine.

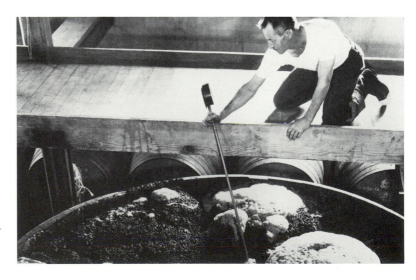

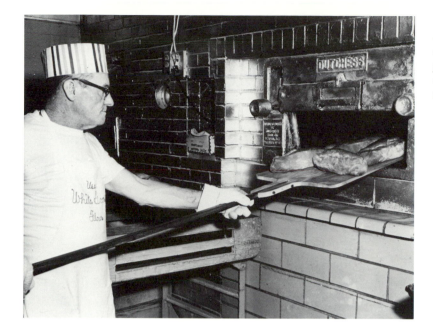

Yeasts ferment the sugars found in most bread doughs. This process produces carbon dioxide, which makes the dough rise.

teria release acids that give the cheeses their distinctive flavor.

Another example of how germs assist in food production is the way yeasts are used to make most breads. Yeasts ferment the sugars in the bread dough. This chemical process produces carbon dioxide gas as a by-product. In the oven, the gas expands, forcing the bread to rise.

Beer and ale brewers use yeasts in a different way. These beverages are made from grain starches, which the germs have trouble breaking down. Brewers begin by allowing the grains to sprout. Then they dry the grains and grind them into a product called malt. Malt contains substances that break down the starches. When yeast is added, the malt ferments, producing beer.

Vinegar is another product made by yeast fermentation. To produce vinegar, wine is purposely exposed to the air. The oxygen in the air causes a chemical reaction in the wine, changing most of the alcohol to acetic acid. Basically, vinegar is sour wine containing little or no alcohol.

Many other foods are produced by using bacteria to cause fermentation. These include sauerkraut, pickles, olives, vanilla, and soy sauce. In the production of soy sauce, for example, soybeans and wheat are mixed together, crushed, and then cooked. Special bacterial cultures are then added, and the mixture is allowed to ferment.

Germs in the oceans and the soil and on animals and people are essential elements of the natural environment. Without these germs, the world would not work the way it does. Human beings have learned to use some of these germs to their advantage, as in the use of bacterial and yeast cultures to aid food production. Unfortunately, people have also learned to use germs for destructive purposes, especially warfare.

Using Germs as a Weapon

All through the twentieth century, scientists and doctors labored to find ways of fighting the germs that cause fatal diseases. Their goal was to stop the spread of disease. But a few scientists had a completely different goal. They sought ways to inflict disease on their country's enemies. The idea is a simple one. Since disease germs can kill, they can be used as a weapon if they can be harnessed. This use of germs is known as germ warfare or biological warfare, referring to the fact that germs are biological agents.

Biological warfare has never been used on a large scale. But germs have been used purposely to kill people, animals, and crops in many isolated incidents. Many of these events occurred in modern times, although earlier societies also used germs to kill people. The difference between then and now is that we know today how and why germs kill. Ancient people did not. They only knew that they could weaken or wipe out their enemies by spreading disease.

Early Biological Warfare Tactics

Although the ancients did not know that germs cause disease, they knew by simple observation that diseases often spread through physical contact. Sometimes,

European settlers battle Native Americans during the colonization of the New World. Some colonists used the deadly smallpox disease as a weapon against the Indians.

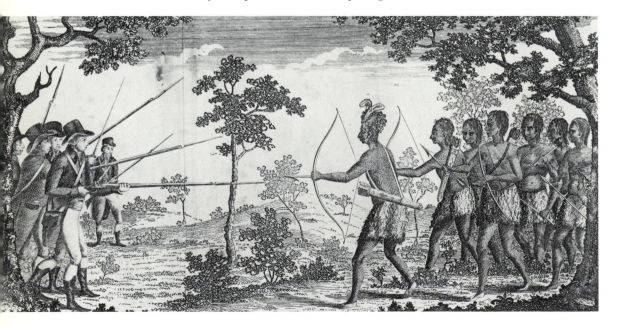

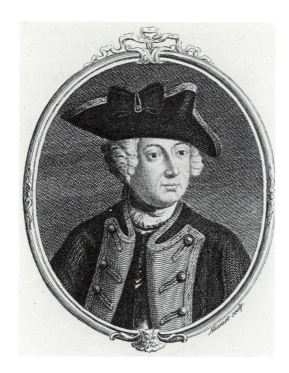

Jeffrey Amherst, a British military officer, ordered troops to give smallpox-infected blankets to North American Indians.

these people put the diseased corpses of animals and humans in wells and other sources of drinking water to contaminate the water and kill their enemies. Another common tactic was to hurl diseased bodies into walled forts and cities that were under siege, hoping the bodies would spread the disease. This occurred in 1347 during the siege of the Italian colony of Kaffa, on the northern coast of the Black Sea. The colony was under siege by the Mongols, who catapulted bodies of bubonic plague victims into the city. Thousands of people in the city contracted the plague, and the Italians surrendered. The incident also had catastrophic consequences for millions of people in distant lands. After the fall of Kaffa, Italian ships carried the plague back to Europe, where the disease wiped out one-third of the con-

tinent's population.

Smallpox was another deadly malady that was used as a weapon. It was used against the Indians of North America a number of times during the centuries of European colonization. During the Indian Wars of the 1700s, for example, Jeffrey Amherst, a British military officer, knowingly gave unwashed blankets used by smallpox victims to Indians in the American colonies. Thousands of Native Americans contracted the disease and died.

The First Experiments with Germ Weapons

In the late 1800s and early 1900s, as serious experimental work in microbiology progressed, many scientists and government officials recognized the potential of germs as weapons. The use of such weapons was and still is generally considered inhumane. For this reason, government-sponsored research into biological weapons was kept secret. It is difficult to say with certainty which countries were doing the research and which were not.

The Germans had the most advanced germ research labs at the time, and many experts suspected them of working on biological weapons. In the early 1900s, officials in the United States and Great Britain accused the Germans of developing biological weapons. The Germans denied these accusations. During World War I, rumors spread that the Germans had infected horses with anthrax and glanders, another animal disease. According to British and French informants, these Germans let the horses loose in France, hoping they would spread the diseases to French animals.

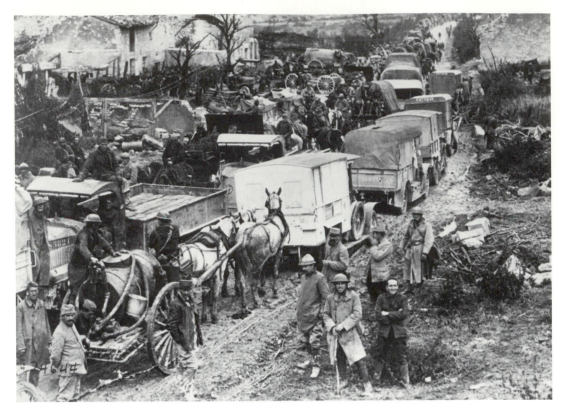

During World War I, the Allies used horses and other animals to transport supplies to the front lines. Rumors spread that the Germans tried to cripple Allied forces by infecting these animals with anthrax.

These rumors were never confirmed.

By the early 1920s, officials in many countries were concerned about the possible development of biological weapons. Such weapons had the potential to infect millions of people with incurable diseases. Great Britain's Winston Churchill had heard reports of biological weapons research going on in many countries. In 1925, he worried about "pestilences [contagious diseases] methodically prepared and deliberately launched upon man and beast . . . Blight to destroy crops, Anthrax to slay horses and cattle, Plague to poison not only armies but whole districts—such are the lines along which military science is remorselessly advancing."

Churchill's reference to anthrax was significant. Scientists and government leaders knew that the disease could kill people as well as animals. People who handled contaminated animals often got skin ulcers and blood poisoning. There were cases of humans inhaling the bacteria, developing choking coughs and fevers, then dying. Government intelligence reports done by various countries at the time indicated that much of the secret biological weapons research being done around the world involved anthrax.

Because of these fears, a clause about germ weapons was included in the 1925 Geneva Protocol. This was an international treaty opposing the use of weapons of mass destruction. The document called for banning "bacterial methods of warfare." Although no countries at the time admitted to having such methods, several nations, including the United States, refused to sign the protocol. The United States finally ratified it in 1974.

Unfortunately, the Geneva Protocol ended up encouraging rather than discouraging research into biological weapons. The signing of such a treaty by so many nations led some governments to suspect that the research was more widespread than previously thought. Fearing that his country might be left out, a Japanese army major named Shiro Ishii toured many of the Euro-pean microbiology labs and other scientific facilities. He became convinced that his country would benefit from the use of germs as a weapon. In 1935, Ishii persuaded the Japanese government to begin a secret biological weapons program.

Great Britain's Winston Churchill was concerned about the use of contagious disease as a wartime weapon.

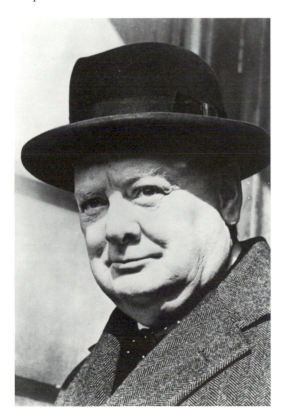

The Japanese Conduct Tests on Humans

By 1939, the Japanese had completed the world's first biological warfare installation. It was located in a remote area of Manchuria, which the Japanese had recently taken from the Chinese and now occupied. Some three thousand scientists and technicians worked at the top secret complex, which had its own school, hospital, and air base. The deadly or disabling diseases studied and grown in cultures at the installation included typhus, anthrax, cholera, bubonic plague, tetanus, smallpox, botulism, tick encephalitis, and tuberculosis. The labs had the capability of producing up to eight tons of bacteria per month. The facility attempted to develop an "anthrax bomb" and exploded two thousand such bombs in lab experiments.

But Ishii wanted to do more than lab research. His country was at war with other Asian nations, and he knew it would only be a matter of time before Japan went to war with the United States and its allies. He wanted to perfect his biological weapons so that Japan could use them in actual warfare. This meant that the weapons would need to be tested on human beings.

Beginning in the early 1940s, Japan's biological facility began tests on human subjects. The Japanese chose prisoners of war, mostly Chinese but also some Americans, British, and Australians. The prisoners were fed food containing cultures of botulism to see how long it would take them to die. In another gruesome experiment, prisoners were tied to stakes and exposed to a bomb containing gas gangrene germs. One witness later said: "The prisoners' heads were covered with metal helmets, and their bodies with screens . . . only the naked buttocks being exposed." The bomb exploded, wounding the men with contaminated metal fragments. All of these victims died from gas gangrene within a few days. The Japanese also injected subjects with anthrax, cholera, bubonic plague, and many other diseases.

While these tests went on at the complex, technicians conducted experiments in the field. Chinese officials reported that Japanese planes flew low over Chinese villages and dropped bags of rice and wheat mixed with fleas. The fleas had been infected with bubonic plague. It is not certain how many Chinese actually died during the experiment, but Chinese officials recorded more than seven hundred plague deaths.

A Biological Arms Race

Japan was not the only nation to develop biological weapons. During the 1930s and 1940s, Great Britain, the Soviet Union, and the United States also launched biological weapons programs. Each country, convinced that its enemies might be making such weapons, raced to develop its own capabilities.

The British feared that Germany would use biological weapons against them, and so they spent a great deal of money on their own program. Like researchers in other countries, the British continued to explore the possibilities of using anthrax. Sometimes, the experiments backfired. In 1942, for example, British researchers exploded their own anthrax bomb near a herd of sheep on the Scottish island of Gruinard. Afterward, they buried the sheep by using a

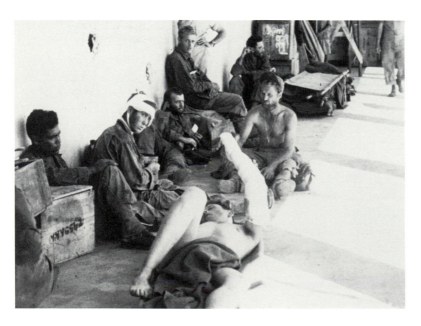

During World War II, the Japanese fed some prisoners of war food containing cultures of botulism to see how long it would take them to die. Here, newly freed American prisoners await transfer to a U.S. hospital.

conventional bomb to start a landslide. But the bomb blew one of the corpses into the sea. The dead sheep floated to the coast of Scotland, where many local animals contracted anthrax. Later, a Scandinavian couple accidentally landed on the island after misreading their sailing charts. The people and their dog contracted anthrax and died.

Over the course of decades, British decontamination experts regularly explored the island, testing to see if the anthrax spores were still dangerous. By the late 1970s, the experts concluded that about 3 or 4 acres of Gruinard's 550 acres were still contaminated. In 1986, scientists used a mixture of chemicals and seawater to kill the remaining spores. Although British officials say the island is now safe, people on the nearby Scottish coast still refer to Gruinard as Anthrax Island.

Experiments with Bubonic Plague

During the 1940s, the Soviets, like the Japanese, sometimes used human subjects. In 1941, the Soviets conducted experiments on political prisoners in Mongolia. According to an intelligence expert who investigated the tests, "The prisoners in chains were brought into an 8-man tent, on the floor of which under wire nets were kept rats infested with pest fleas; the latter transmit the infection to the subject of the experiment. The experiments were positive in most cases and the infection ended in bubonic plague." Some of the prisoners escaped and infected nearby Mongolian villages. Reportedly, between three and five thousand people died of the plague.

Between 1942 and 1945, the United States invested more than $40 million in biological weapons research. A large portion of this money went into building a weapons plant in Vigo, Indiana. The plant had the capability of producing up to one million biological bombs per month. In 1944 and 1945, German and Japanese officials accused the United States of dropping biological crop-killing bombs on their countries. These charges were never proven. At the end of the war, the government sold the Vigo plant to a medicines manufacturer. But U.S. biological weapons research continued, as it did in Great Britain, the Soviet Union, and other countries.

The Modern Biological Threat

In the post-World War II years, knowledge of germs increased. With the invention of even more powerful micro-

In 1969, President Richard Nixon ordered all U.S. biological weapons destroyed.

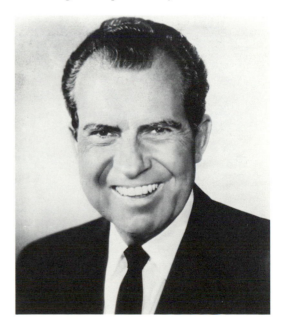

scopes came better understanding of viruses and their potential as lethal weapons. Biological warfare specialists began to work with such viral diseases as Rocky Mountain spotted fever, dengue fever, and Rift Valley fever. The planes, missiles, and other devices that could be used to deliver biological weapons to their targets also became more sophisticated.

Banning Biological Weapons

By the 1960s, scientists and military experts in many countries warned that a biological war was a real possibility. They said that such a war might wipe out large segments of humanity. Government leaders around the world came under increasing pressure to eliminate this threat. In 1969, President Richard Nixon ordered all U.S. biological weapons destroyed. Soon afterward, on April 10, 1972, the United States, Soviet Union, and eighty-five other countries signed the Biological Warfare Convention. This agreement, which was ratified by the United Nations, banned the use of biological weapons in war.

But the agreement did not end the threat of biological weapons. Although it prohibited the use of such weapons, it did not prohibit research. The United States insisted that the Soviet Union was

U.S. Air Force members cheer as an F-16 departs for a bombing mission in Iraq. U.S. planes destroyed Iraqi biological weapons plants during the many bombing missions of the Persian Gulf War.

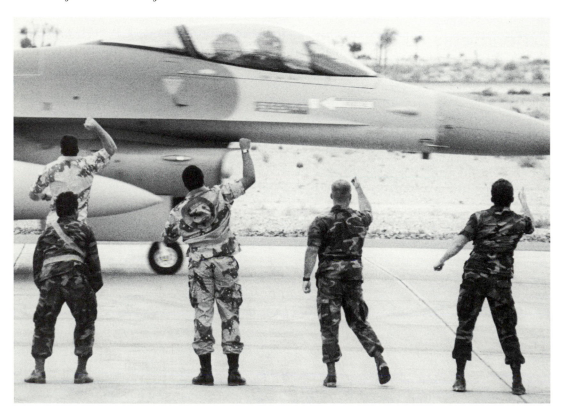

continuing to study the military use of germs. The Soviets denied this, but an incident in 1979 proved the charge was accurate. An accident at a biological weapons factory in the Soviet town of Sverdlovsk released deadly anthrax spores, killing hundreds of people and injuring thousands more. According to Soviet witnesses, medical authorities burned the bodies of the dead, and bull-dozers stripped away the contaminated topsoil.

In addition to the threat of biological weapons from individual nations, there is also a growing threat from terrorist groups. Some of these groups have attempted to manufacture their own devices. In 1974, for example, a group of forty-eight Italians was arrested on charges that it had purposely placed cholera cultures in Italian public water sources in 1973. And in 1980, French police found evidence that the Red Army Faction, a German terrorist organization, was working on biological devices. The terrorists were making botulin toxin, a poison given off by bacteria, in a bathtub in a French apartment.

Many people around the world worry about possible future uses of biological weapons. More and more nations appear to be acquiring the knowledge and technology needed to develop

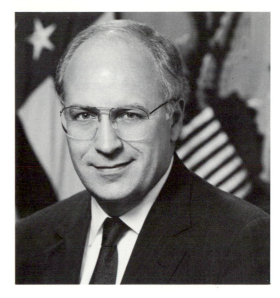

According to U.S. Secretary of Defense Dick Cheney, at least ten countries will have the capability of using biological weapons by the year 2000.

them. Iraq, for instance, developed biological weapons capabilities before U.S. planes destroyed its research labs and weapons plants during the 1991 Persian Gulf War. According to Secretary of Defense Dick Cheney, by the year 2000, at least ten nations will have biological weapons and the equipment to use them. Ensuring that these terrible weapons are never used will be one of the most important challenges faced by world leaders in the twenty-first century.

Finding New Uses for Germs

In the twentieth century, scientists have discovered many innovative ways to use germs to make people's lives better. Germs are regularly used to treat sewage and to control insects, and they are also used in the mining of uranium and copper. In addition, researchers are experimenting with using germs to clean up disastrous oil spills. In other experiments, germs are being tested on plants and crops to make them more resistant to disease. Scientists are constantly working to improve and expand these and other germ-based technologies.

Germs in Sewage Treatment

Sewage is the mixture of water and solid waste materials that people routinely discard each day. Sewage includes all of the substances that go down toilets as well as through bathtub, sink, and street drains. The solid parts of sewage make up less than one-tenth of 1 percent of the total. The rest is water. Yet, in a large city, as many as one thousand tons of these solid materials, called sludge, can build up in a single day. Scientists and engineers regularly treat, or purify, these wastes before disposing of them.

Germs play a primary role in modern sewage treatment. Certain germs in the environment feed on and digest sludge, turning much of it into harmless substances such as water, carbon dioxide, and various alcohols. Nearly all major cities in the United States now have sewage treatment facilities where germs have been added on a large scale to purify wastes. Unfortunately, this is not the case in most other countries. For instance, more than 80 percent of the 125

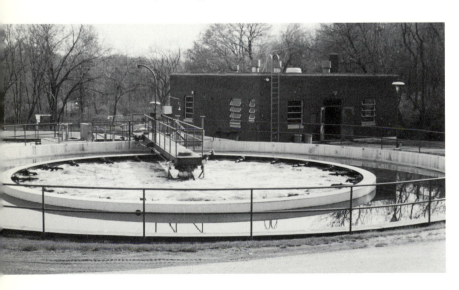

Germs play an important role in sewage treatment. Some germs digest sludge, transforming much of it into harmless substances.

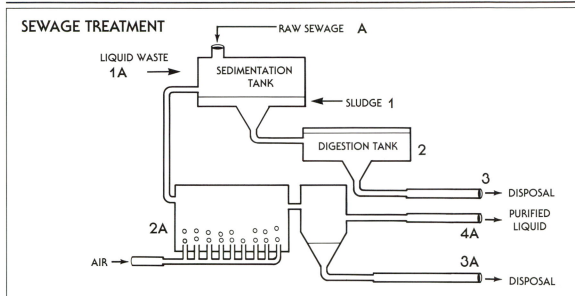

SEWAGE TREATMENT

RAW SEWAGE   **A**

LIQUID WASTE
1A

SEDIMENTATION TANK

SLUDGE 1

DIGESTION TANK   2

3   DISPOSAL

PURIFIED LIQUID

2A

4A

AIR

3A   DISPOSAL

New uses for germs are being found everyday. One of the most promising is the use of germs to treat sewage, turning much of it into harmless substances such as water and carbon dioxide.

Since different types of germs are used in this process, it is necessary to separate the solid waste, or sludge, from the liquid waste. The two types of waste are then treated differently.

(A) Sludge: Raw sewage is pumped into a sedimentation tank, where the sludge settles to the bottom of the tank. Here, special germs begin to digest it (1). The sludge is then pumped into a special digestion tank, where still other germs continue to break it down (2). The digested sludge is no longer toxic and is removed for disposal (3). Some of it is dried, sterilized, and then used as fertilizer for gardens and farms.

(B) Liquid waste: Liquid waste is separated from solid waste (1A). The liquid is exposed to air (2A). This process, called aeration, speeds the growth of specific kinds of germs. These germs digest small solid waste products floating in the water. The digested solid waste is removed for disposal (3A). The remaining liquid is pure enough to release into an ocean or river without polluting it (4A).

largest cities located along the coasts of the Mediterranean Sea release untreated sewage directly into the sea.

The first step in modern sewage treatment, called primary treatment, separates the sludge from the liquid components of the sewage. The raw sewage is pumped into large open tanks, where the solid materials slowly settle to the bottom. During this process, germs begin to digest some of the sludge.

The next phase, called secondary treatment, is usually accomplished in two steps. In the first, the liquid portion of the sewage is aerated, or exposed to large amounts of air. The oxygen in the air encourages specific germs to grow quickly and digest particles of waste floating in the water. In the second step of secondary treatment, the solid wastes are pumped into special tanks. There, other kinds of germs digest and break down the sludge. One by-product created by this digestion is methane, a burnable gas. Many sewage treatment plants capture the methane as it is released and use it as a fuel to help run their machinery.

Scientists are constantly working to produce new strains of bacteria and other germs that will digest sewage more efficiently. One new process is called tertiary treatment. It combines germs and chemicals to purify liquid wastes so thoroughly that they can be recycled as drinking water. Presently, this is a costly process, but wastewater treated in this manner is already being used to irrigate crops in many areas of the United States.

Germs Used to Fight Insect Pests

Many insects carry dangerous disease germs, while others cause serious damage to crops each year. Scientists are always searching for ways to eliminate these insect pests. In the twentieth century, most insecticides, substances that kill insects, have been chemical sprays. Chemical agents such as DDT effectively kill insects, but these chemicals often remain in the soil as toxic pollutants. These toxins eventually enter streams and poison fish and other food sources used by animals and people.

As an alternative, germs can be used to kill insect pests without causing environmental pollution. The German scientist G.S. Berliner first proposed the idea in the early 1900s. Berliner noticed that certain kinds of bacteria destroyed moth caterpillars, which destroy crops. But the way the bacteria did this was not well understood at the time, and the idea was largely forgotten until the 1970s and 1980s.

Scientists eventually learned that the bacteria Berliner observed produce highly poisonous substances during reproduction. These poisons accumulate on plant leaves and are ingested by the

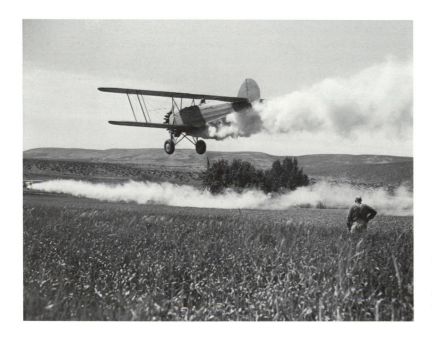

Germs can be used to control the insects that destroy crops. However, many farmers still protect their crops by spraying chemical insecticides.

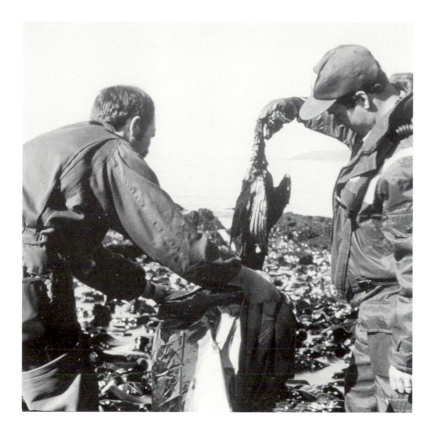

Some kinds of germs have been used to help clean up oil spills.

caterpillars of moths, butterflies, and related insects. Once inside the digestive tract, or gut, of a caterpillar, the poisons dissolve the gut walls. The insect soon becomes paralyzed and dies.

To make the germ-based insecticide, scientists grow large cultures of bacteria and harvest them at the time when they are producing the poisons. The bacteria are dried and made into a powder that can be dusted on crops by ground-based machines or airplanes. Pests such as tomato hornworms, gypsy moth caterpillars, alfalfa caterpillars, and cabbage worms are regularly controlled using this method.

An important advantage of germ insecticides is that they appear not to affect plants and other animals. The poisons break down quickly into harmless substances and do not accumulate in the soil, which makes this method environmentally safe. Farmers have reported such a high rate of success with this approach that scientists are experimenting with bacteria that might be used to kill other kinds of insect pests.

Germs That Eat Oil

Scientists have long known that certain kinds of germs consume petroleum, or oil. The germs break down the oil into simpler, harmless substances, a process known as biodegradation. This process occurs constantly in nature but happens randomly and very slowly, so it does not have much immediate impact on large oil spills.

It was not until the 1980s that researchers seriously considered creating

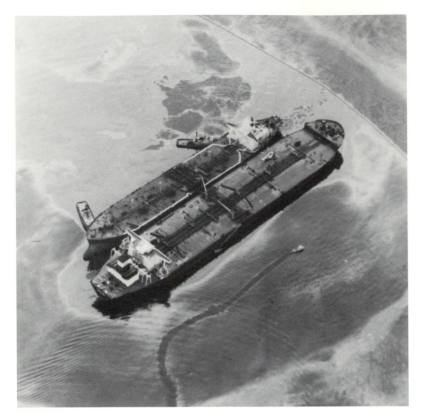

The Exxon Baton Rouge *unloaded oil from the* Exxon Valdez *after it ran aground in Alaska in 1989. Later, researchers grew oil-consuming bacteria in bags of fertilizer. They deposited these bags on the beaches and inlets of Prince William Sound, the site of the spill.*

concentrated batches of germs to fight oil spills. There were several reasons why this technique was not tried sooner. For one thing, scientists were not sure how these germs could be delivered effectively into a spill. Just sprinkling them onto an oil slick would not work because the action of waves and currents quickly disperse the germs. There was also the problem of having the germs ready at the right time and in the right place. Oil spills are usually accidental, and so their location cannot be predicted.

The first major use of germs to fight a big oil spill occurred in 1989. The oil tanker *Exxon Valdez* hit a reef in Prince William Sound in Alaska, spilling millions of gallons of crude petroleum. The oil fouled hundreds of miles of beaches and killed thousands of birds, otters, and other animals. Conventional cleanup methods could remove only some of the oil, and scientists decided to test the newest germ techniques.

The researchers grew large masses of oil-consuming bacteria in sacks of fertilizer. They placed some of these sacks at preplanned positions on the bottom of inlets in Prince William Sound. They placed other sacks containing bacteria on about seventy miles of beaches lining the sound. The plan was that the action of waves and tides would flush through the fertilizer and carry the bacteria directly into the oil slick. There, the tiny organisms would begin to biodegrade the oil.

Researchers have reported some initial successes with the germ technique. Studies made during the first two years of bacteria use in Prince William Sound show that the method is effective when

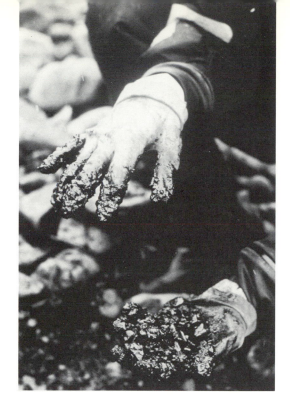

The major drawback of using oil-consuming bacteria to clean up spills is that the process is slow. It takes two to five years to reduce the amount of oil from a large oil spill.

combined with other cleanup methods. The germ technique was used experimentally in cleanups of several other spills in 1990 and 1991. The major draw-

back of this method is that it works very slowly. Two to five years are needed to significantly reduce the amount of oil in a large spill. Scientists are currently attempting to grow new strains of bacteria that eat oil faster, and the technique shows much promise for the future.

Other Modern Uses for Germs

Each year, modern science finds new ways to use germs productively. Some of these uses, like cleaning up oil spills, are human refinements of already existing natural processes. Another such example is the use of germs in mining technology. During the thousands of years that copper has been mined, miners were unaware that the mining process was aided by germs. Scientists discovered this phenomenon in 1957. At that time, they learned that the mining process would be impossible without the actions of certain "rock-eating" bacteria. The bacteria, called *Thiobacillus ferrooxidans*, consume the rust that forms in de-

In a copper mine, Thiobacillus ferrooxidans *cause chemical reactions to occur in the copper-laden rock. One of the reactions separates the copper from the other elements found in the rock.*

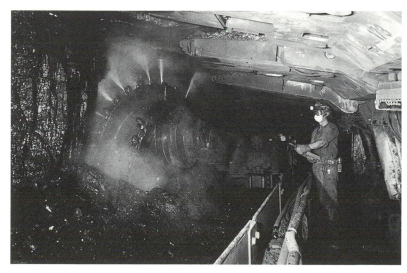

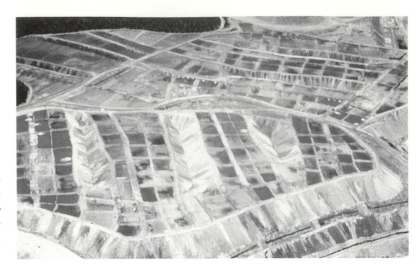

An aerial view of dumps in which rocks containing copper are concentrated in ponds with Thiobacillus ferrooxidans.

posits of iron and sulfur. Armed with this knowledge, mining engineers have significantly improved copper-mining technology.

The engineers grind up rocks containing copper and other minerals and throw them into a pit called a dump. The *thiobacillus* bacteria already exist in these rocks and multiply in the dump. The engineers pour a mixture of water and a powerful acid, called a leach solution, into the dump. As the leach solution circulates through the copper-bearing rocks in the dump, the bacteria cause certain chemical reactions to take place. One of these reactions separates the copper from the iron, sulfur, and other minerals in the rocks. Engineers have learned to use similar processes utilizing different bacteria for extracting manganese, uranium, and other metals from rocks.

While germs offer great promise in the environment, scientists have also

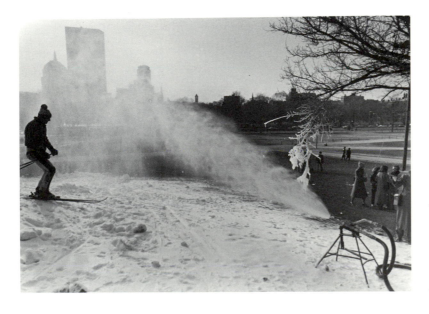

One genetically manufactured germ produces a protein that makes water freeze at higher-than-normal temperatures. This germ is used to make artificial snow at some U.S. and European ski resorts.

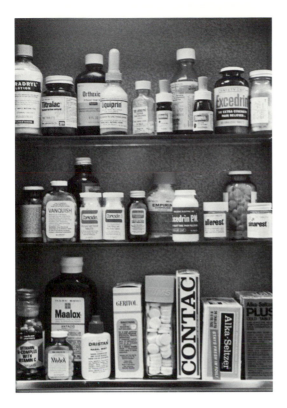

made efforts toward finding new ways of using germs to benefit daily human life. The world's population is rising steadily, and new sources of protein are increasingly in demand. Using germs to produce protein may be one way of meeting that demand. Protein makes up about 50 percent of the body tissues of animals and people and is an essential part of any diet. Meats, dairy products, vegetables, and fruits all contain various types of proteins. Scientists have learned to mix certain germs with carbon-rich materials such as alcohol, petroleum, and wood pulp in order to produce crude proteins. As the germs consume these materials, chemical reactions take place that produce these proteins. Germs reproduce very quickly, and a culture can double in weight in a few hours and sometimes in an hour or less. Therefore, this method can make large quantities of protein in a short amount of time. Proteins produced in

Today, scientists are producing new kinds of drugs and medicines from germ cultures.

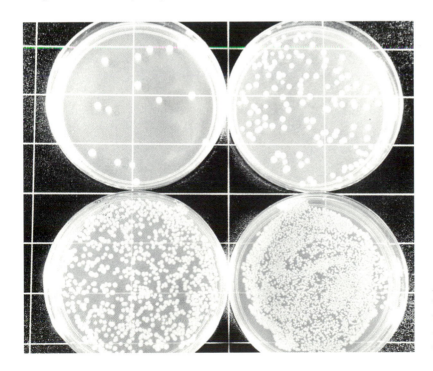

Bacteria cultures in various stages of reproduction. A culture can double in weight in a few hours or less.

this way are not yet widely used by humans, but many animal feeds are currently made by mixing germs and alcohol.

Other modern uses for germs are the result of innovative technologies created by human beings. For instance, scientists have invented new ways to make many medicines and drugs from germ cultures. Germs are routinely used to produce steroids, which promote muscle growth, and birth control pills.

The newest germ technology involves genetic engineering. Genetic engineering is the manipulation of genes, the tiny elements within cells that carry the blueprints of life, in order to change the way in which an organism will develop. Scientists are finding ways to change these genetic blueprints in germs. The goal is to create totally new strains of germs that will have certain improved characteristics. For instance, a manufactured germ strain might be able to eat more oil than a naturally existing strain.

Already, genetically manufactured germs are being used in a wide range of products. One new germ makes plants and crops more resistant to disease. Other new germs are used in the production of artificial skin to heal burns and other wounds. Genetic engineering of germs is also used in recreational products. One new germ, for example, produces a protein that makes water freeze at higher-than-normal temperatures. This is currently being used to create artificial snow at ski resorts in the United States and Europe.

There is no doubt that as new and better lab instruments and techniques are discovered, knowledge about germs will increase. People will continue to find novel ways to use germs to improve the quality of human life. Eventually, it may even be possible to completely eliminate or control the germs that cause disease. But there is still much to learn. The oldest and simplest of nature's creatures have not yet given up all their secrets to the people who peer at them through the lenses of microscopes.

Glossary

■ ■

aerate: To expose something to the air.

animalcules: Term used in the 1600s by Antonie van Leeuwenhoek to describe the tiny creatures now known as germs.

antibodies: Substances manufactured by the body to attack foreign substances, including germs.

antiseptic: A germ-killing substance.

biodegradation: The process by which microorganisms digest various materials, including oil, by chemically breaking them down into simpler substances.

biogenesis: The concept that all living cells originate from preexisting living cells.

biological warfare: The use of germs as weapons.

cell: The basic unit of living matter from which all plants and animals are built.

coma: Deep, prolonged unconciousness caused by disease or injury.

contagious: Diseases that easily spread from person to person through contact.

contaminate: To soil, stain, or infect by contact or association.

culture: Growth of living material such as bacteria in a prepared substance.

decay: To rot or decompose.

epidemic: A widespread outbreak of a disease.

epidemiology: The science that deals with how diseases are transmitted and spread.

fermentation: A process by which germs cause chemical changes in foods and beverages, as in the transformation of grape juice into wine.

fission: A splitting apart; the method by which bacteria reproduce, dividing in half.

genetic engineering: The manipulation of genetic material, which is reponsible for transmission of characteristics from parent to offspring.

germs: The general name given to microscopic living things, including bacteria, fungi, algae, protozoa, and viruses.

germ theory: The concept that germs cause disease.

infect: To contaminate with a disease-producing substance or agent.

influenza: An acute, highly contagious viral disease commonly known as flu.

insecticide: A substance that kills insects.

leach solution: A mixture of water and acid used to speed chemical processes that assist in mining.

microbiology: The study of microorganisms.

mucus: A fluid secreted in warm, moist areas of the body.

mutate: To undergo a major physical or biochemical change in some inheritable characteristic.

nucleus: The central part of a cell.

nutrient: A substance that provides nourishment.

organism: Any living thing.

pasteurization: The process that uses heat to kill dangerous germs in beverages such as milk and wine.

plague: Any deadly epidemic disease.

primary sewage treatment: The process that allows solids in sewage to settle.

protein: Complex, naturally occurring substances found in all living organisms.

secondary sewage treatment: The process in which microorganisms digest sewage wastes.

sludge: The solid components of sewage.

spontaneous generation: The theory, disproved in the 1800s, that living things, including germs, come into existence randomly from nonliving materials.

spore: A tiny, single- or multi-celled body produced during the process of reproduction of many plants; capable of giving rise to a new individual.

symbiosis: A relationship in which two living things benefit from living together.

toxic: Poisonous.

For Further Reading

Nathan Aaseng, *The Disease Fighters*. Minneapolis,
MN: Lerner Publications, 1987.

Thomas G. Aylesworth, *The World of Microbes*. New
York: Franklin Watts, 1975.

Melvin Berger, *The Disease Detectives*. New York:
Thomas Y. Crowell, 1978.

Timothy Levi Biel, *The Black Death*. San Diego, CA:
Lucent Books, 1989.

Parnell Donahue and Helen Capellaro, *Germs
Make Me Sick*. New York: Alfred A. Knopf, 1975.

Daniel N. Lapedes, *Helpful Microorganisms*. New
York: The World Publishing Company, 1968.

Don Nardo, *Oil Spills*. San Diego, CA: Lucent
Books, 1991.

L.B. Taylor, *Chemical and Biological Warfare*. New
York: Franklin Watts, 1985.

Marianne and Mary-Alice Tully, *Dread Diseases*. New
York: Franklin Watts, 1978.

Works Consulted

I. Edward Alcamo, *Fundamentals of Microbiology.* Reading, MA: Addison-Wesley, 1983.

Joseph D. Douglass Jr. and Neil C. Livingstone, *America the Vulnerable: The Threat of Chemical/Biological Warfare.* Lexington, MA: D.C. Heath, 1987.

Great Disasters: Dramatic Stories of Nature's Awesome Powers. Pleasantville, NY: Reader's Digest Association, 1989.

W.E. Gutman, "A Poison in Every Caldron," *Omni,* February 1991.

Robert Harris and Jeremy Paxman, *A Higher Form Of Killing: The Secret Story of Chemical and Biological Warfare.* New York: Hill & Wang, 1982.

Robert P. Hudson, *Disease and Its Control: The Shaping of Modern Thought.* Westport, CT: Greenwood Press, 1983.

Peter Jaret, "The Disease Detectives," *National Geographic,* January 1991.

Ernest A. Meyer, *Microorganisms and Human Disease.* New York: Prentice-Hall, 1974.

Theodor Rosebury, *Life on Man.* New York: Viking, 1969.

Jay Stuller, "Cleanliness Has Only Recently Become a Virtue," *Smithsonian,* February 1991.

Gerard J. Tortora, et al., *Microbiology: An Introduction.* New York: Benjamin/Cummings, 1989.

Index

About the Author

▪ ▪

Don Nardo is an actor, film director, and composer, as well as an award-winning writer. As an actor, he has appeared in more than fifty stage productions. He has also worked before or behind the camera in twenty films. Several of his musical compositions, including a young person's version of *The War of the Worlds* and the oratorio *Richard III,* have been played by regional orchestras. Mr. Nardo's writing credits include short stories, articles, and more than twenty books, including *Lasers: Humanity's Magic Light; Anxiety and Phobias; The Irish Potato Famine; Exercise; Gravity: The Universal Force;* and *The Mexican - American War.* Among his other writings are an episode of ABC's "Spenser: For Hire" and numerous screenplays. Mr. Nardo lives with his wife, Christine, on Cape Cod, Massachusetts.

Picture Credits

■ ■